Helping Hurting People

Helping Hurting People

A Team Approach to Caring for the Whole Person
A Training Manual for Spiritual Caregivers

*Peace of mind makes the body strong
Envy makes the body sick.
Proverbs 14 : 30*

Dan Fountain, M.D., MPH
King College, Bristol TN

Sherry O'Donnell, D.O.
Rappha Medical Clinic
St. Joseph MI

All Scripture quotations unless otherwise marked are taken from the Good News Translation - Second Edition, Copyright 1992 by American Bible Society. Used by Permission.

Scripture quotations marked (NIV) are taken from the New International Version ® of the Holy Bible. Copyright © 1973, 1978, 1984 by International Bible Society Used by permission of Zondervan Publishing House. All rights reserved.

Copyright © 2008 by Daniel E. Fountain, M.D. All rights reserved.

Printed in the United States of America

Publishing services by Selah Publishing Group, LLC, Tennessee. The views expressed or implied in this work do not necessarily reflect those of Selah Publishing Group.

No part of this publication may be reproduced, stored in a retrieval system or transmitted in any way by any means, electronic, mechanical, photocopy, recording or otherwise, without the prior permission of the author except as provided by USA copyright law.

ISBN: 978-1-58930-223-5
Library of Congress Control Number: 2008908075

Dear Sister or Brother,

We want to welcome you to this course on caring for the whole person. We also want to welcome you to the spiritual care team. You likely have chosen this curriculum because you have a desire to help hurting people and you have sensed that God is calling you to this ministry. Likewise, God has called us to this ministry. We will be working together with you, your instructor, and the Lord as you go through these lessons.

This is not an easy ministry. Most people who seek medical attention are struggling with personal issues that cause heavy burdens in their heart. Medical science is increasingly aware that these personal issues and heavy burdens negatively impact wellness. Often they aggravate an existing illness and impede the recovery process. They may even be a primary cause of an illness. Therefore, it is essential that we try to discern what is going on in the life of the person, discover any inner problems they may have, and offer care for those problems. That type of care includes making available to them the wonderful resources Christ and God's Word provide to heal the broken heart and the wounded spirit. The content of this course is about how to establish a caring relationship with sick persons which can enable them to share their real concerns and deal with inner problems. We will discuss how to discern inner issues people may have, and what spiritual resources we can offer them to assist in their recovery.

Goals for this team approach to caring for the whole person are:
1. To train health providers and spiritual caregivers in how, simultaneously, to provide emotional and spiritual care for sick persons.
2. To integrate personal and spiritual care with medical care in the same facility setting.
3. To implement a model of care that will restore wholeness to the practice of medicine.

At the end of this course participants should be able to explain the following:
1. The principles of wholeness both from a biblical and a scientific point of view.
2. The resources that Christ offers for healing the broken heart and the   wounded spirit
3. The principles and practice of a caring relationship
4. A Christ-centered approach in helping people resolve personal life issues
5. How you function effectively as a member of the team delivering whole person healthcare.

Awareness that sick persons have spiritual needs is becoming increasingly measured by accrediting agencies; therefore hospitals and health programs are challenged to develop ways to provide spiritual care. Much of this care, however, is 'generic' spiritual care that simply encourages sick people to use whatever spiritual resources they have to cope better with their illness.

This course offers a specifically Christian approach to caring for emotional and spiritual needs. We have discovered that a personal relationship with Jesus Christ has therapeutic benefits. It brings new meaning and purpose for life, peace and joy to the spirit, and hope for the future. It is our prayer that, through this course, you will learn how those benefits improve the health and healing of people. This is not to say that a person must become a Christian in order to find healing. Even Jesus healed many who did not follow him after they were healed. It does mean, however, that within the Christian faith are particular resources of great benefit for both health and healing.

This is not an easy course for there is much work to be done. There are classes to attend, considerable reading involved, and questions to think about and answer. Please remember that we have a wonderful Teacher, the Spirit of God, who leads us into all truth. We encourage you to approach this training prayerfully, making prayer your habit as you read and as you come to class. As you listen to us, to your instructor, and to your fellow students, be listening also for that inner voice; those deep thoughts that come from God, Himself, through the Spirit. We will be in touch by e-mail with your instructor, so that if difficult questions arise, we will be available to consult with you.

You will discover new truths in God's Word, even in passages with which you are already very familiar. You will see new meanings in them about healing, and find new resources to help hurting people. We think you will find help through this course for your own inner burdens or life issues.. We are ready to be of whatever help we can be to you as the Spirit of God leads us. You will be learning new skills in building relationships and how to come alongside hurting people. You are entering new territory and, just as God told Joshua, "Be strong and of good courage, for the Lord your God is with you wherever you go."

Dan Fountain, M.D.
1805 Turban Court
Fort Myers, FL 33908
e-mail: dfountain2@king.edu

Sherry O'Donnell, D.O.
Rappha Medical Center
3911 Stonegate Park Drive
St. Joseph, MI 49085
e-mail: saodonnell@rappha.com

Contents

1	The Problem of Modern Medicine	9
2	How Have We Gotten into This Mess?	17
3	Jesus as Our Model	23
4	The Biblical Perspective on Wholeness	31
5	The Heart/Body Relationship from the Scientific Perspective	37
6	The Architecture of the Heart	43
7	Heart Problems That Affect Health	51
8	Sin and Its Consequences for Our Health	57
9	Salvation is Not Purification	63
10	What Did Jesus Christ Accomplish for Our Healing?	67
11	Establishing a Caring Relationship	71
12	Personal and Spiritual Assessment	81
13	Taking a Spiritual History	85
14	Praying with Sick Persons	91
15	Doing a Life Review	97
16	Problem of Self-Identity	107
17	Anger, Illness, and Forgiving Others	111
18	Helping People Who Are Carrying a Heavy Load of Stress	119
19	Helping a Person Face Cancer	125
20	Helping a Person Who is Grieving	129
21	Helping People Cope with Bad News and Terminal Illness	133
22	Practical Applications	141
	Bibliography	147

Lesson 1
The Problem of Modern Medicine

Read also: God, Medicine, and Miracles, *chapter one*

Medical science has accomplished many wonderful things. The discovery and implementation of antibiotics, new diagnostic and surgical techniques, and organ transplantation have greatly extended life and improved its quality. Although medicine cannot cure many chronic illnesses, it can manage many of them and enable people to cope better with the aspects of the illness. Yet, for all of its accomplishments, modern medicine is still inadequate in restoring sick persons to wholeness. The focus of medicine is almost entirely on the physical aspects of illnesses. The spiritual and psychosocial wellness of one's health is either denied or considered irrelevant, and the ramifications of this on a person's health is often unrecognized or referred to a specialist in those areas. No one treats the whole person.

Question for reflection: A man with severe heart disease comes to the physician who refers him to you for spiritual care. When you ask him about his faith, he responds angrily: "How can I believe in a God who allowed a drunk driver to kill my little grandson?" How would you respond to him? (*Before proceeding, spend five minutes thinking about this.*)

* * * * * * * * * * *

During the past one hundred years the focus of medicine has changed radically. Formerly, medicine was concerned about people, attempting to heal them when they were ill and restore them to wholeness. The key to good care was the doctor/patient relationship. With the rapid rise of science, the emphasis has changed from the person who is ill to the evidence science provides for care. Every medical intervention has to be scientifically valid. We now practice 'evidence-based medicine,' using only what can be 'proved' scientifically. This is good and has accomplished much. Yet, since psychosocial and spiritual aspects of illness cannot be measured objectively, these elements are ignored by most medical practitioners. The sick person has been reduced to an object to be analyzed and repaired.

In addition, rising costs, increasing litigation, time constraints, and mushrooming demands of medical technology keep medical caregivers from taking the time necessary to listen to the story of sick persons, discern underlying personal problems that may be complicating the illness, and dealing with them appropriately. Hence it is urgent that this team approach to care become a reality, where people are trained as spiritual caregivers to listen to sick persons and provide encouragement, support, and spiritual care.

Chaplaincies now exist in many hospitals to provide personal and spiritual care, and this is a major step forward. At the same time many churches are having 'healing services' to pray for sick persons. This also is a step forward. Yet seldom does this become a truly 'team approach' between medical, psycho-social, and spiritual caregivers, nor do medicine and chaplaincies care for the trinity of humanity. Each still deals with their perceived discipline, and area of training. So a team approach is necessary to provide care for the whole person under one roof and at one time to bring about total health. It is <u>primary care</u> at the entry level, in which a sick person can be evaluated at the first visit to the health professional and cared for <u>as a whole person.</u>

The following diagram shows the divided approach to the care of sick persons

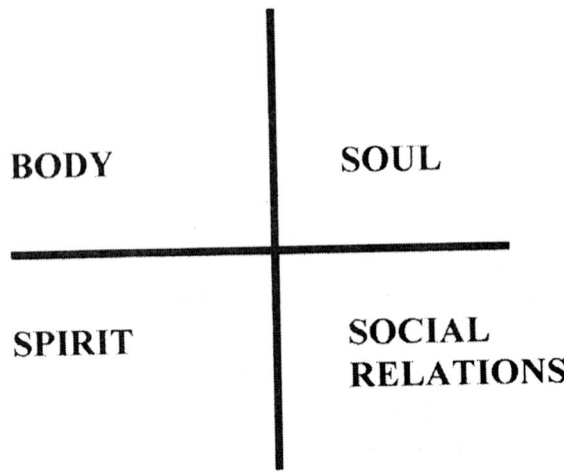

1. The physical body is under the care of health professionals.
2. The soul – thoughts, feelings, emotions – is under the care of counselors, psychologists, or psychiatrists.
3. Spiritual problems are referred to pastors, priests or other religious leaders.
4. Social problems come under the care of trained social workers.

The different aspects of care require separate appointments in separate facilities, with separate costs and billings. Rarely do the caregivers consult each other, or try to integrate their different concerns. There is no <u>team approach</u> to care for the whole person.

It is important to remember that what happens in one dimension of life affects all others. A physical illness impacts the soul, spirit and social aspects of a person's health and may cause fear, depression, or disturbances in the family and other relationships, and thereby further disrupt health.

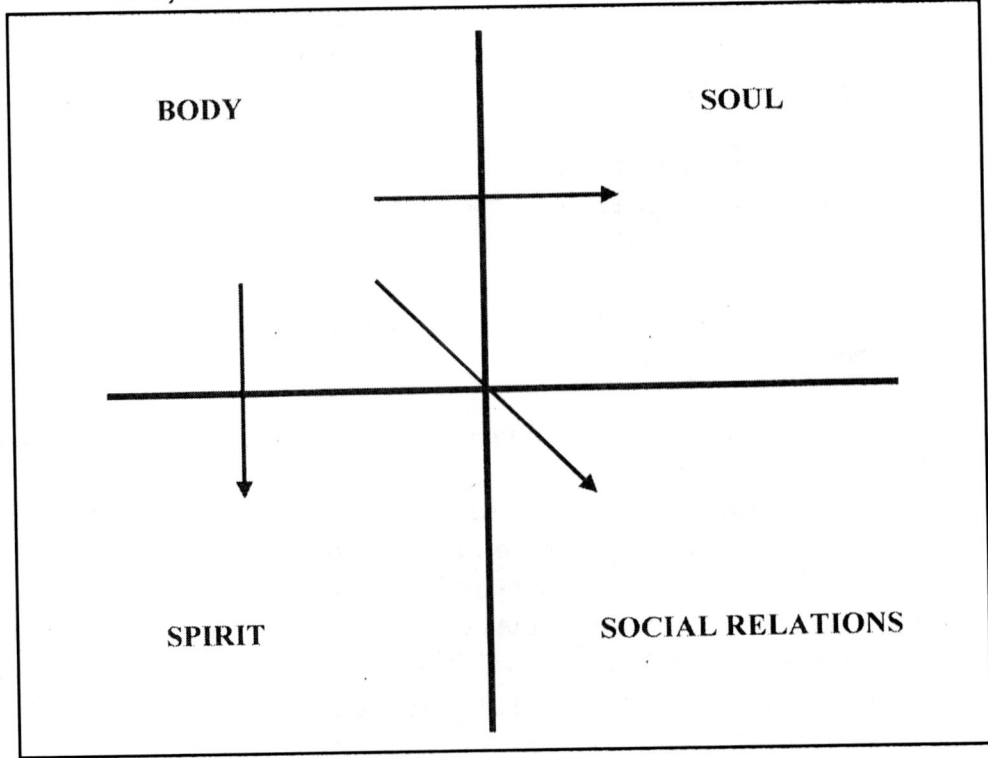

It is likewise true that emotional problems, spiritual malaise, and social conflicts or dysfunctional relationships can affect the other dimensions of life, including the body as we shall see later.

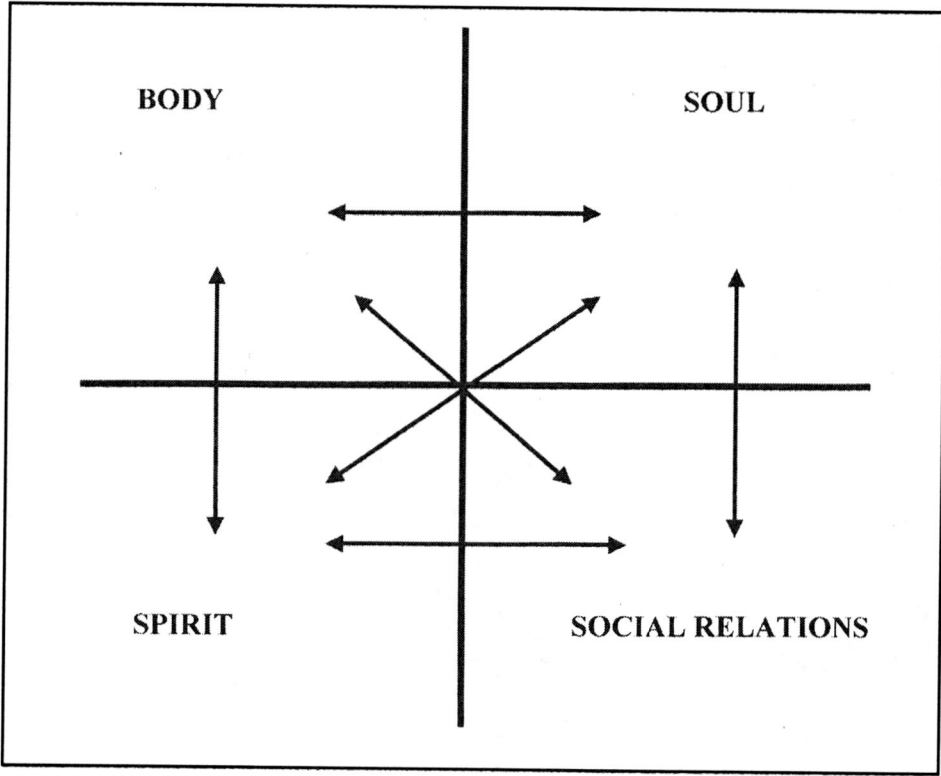

Consider what can go wrong in each of the four dimensions of life:

BODY	SOUL
Hypertension, heart disease	Fear, worries
Chronic pain or inflammation	Anxiety
Auto-immune disorders	Anger, bitterness, resentment
Digestive problems	Shame, guilt
Many infections	Jealousy, envy
Malignancies	Grief
SPIRIT	**SOCIAL RELATIONS**
Poor self-image	Dysfunctional relationships
Depression	Divorce
Meaninglessness	Abuse
Sense of rejection	Poverty
Loneliness	Unemployment

Problems in the soul, spirit, or social realms can affect the physical body in various ways:
1. produce physical symptoms and even illness
2. aggravate existing illness
3. impede recovery from illness

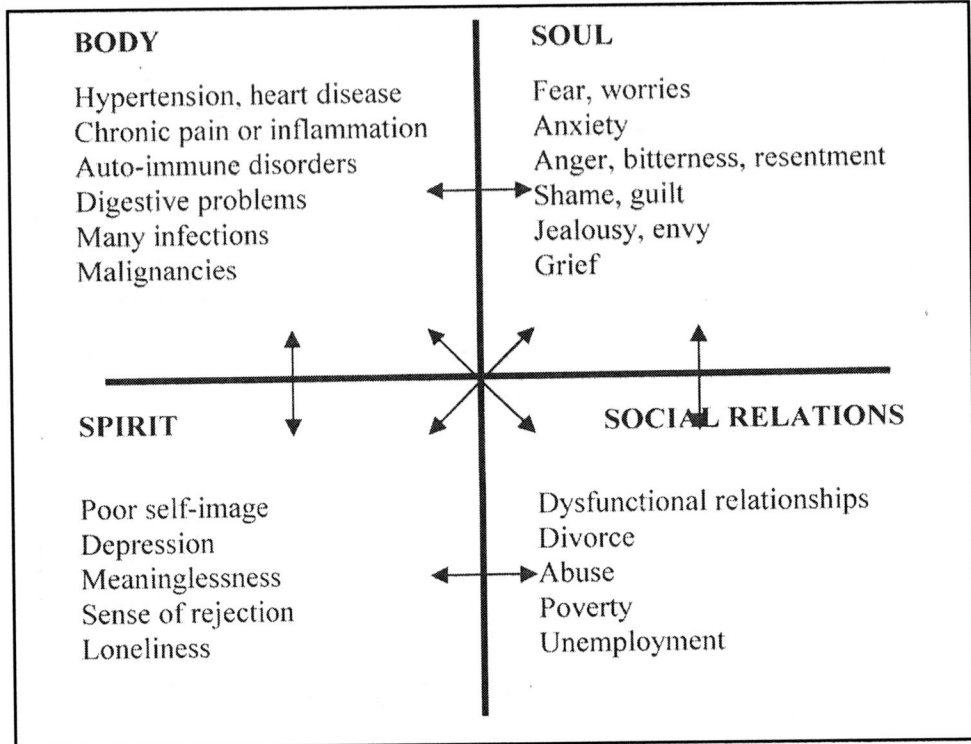

From this, it is clear that unless care is rendered for sick persons as whole persons, we cannot expect to restore them to wholeness. Health practitioners, of course, do not heal people, nor restore people to wholeness. Only God can do that; yet he has chosen to do that through those who work with him as his servants. We have available to us the immense healing power through Jesus Christ and the resources of medicine to make people whole. The Bible and now medical science recognize wholeness as an essential quality of life. We will discuss this in detail as we go further into this study.

A crucial question is: How can this be done? How can we bring together care for all dimensions of life? Can we apply this integrated approach in one clinical setting? The answer to the last question is Yes, and models of this approach now exist. No one person, however, no matter how well trained, can give in-depth care to all dimensions of a person's life or illness. A team approach is essential, and this requires at least four things.

1. People adequately trained to provide care for each dimension of life
2. Training of all of these people to understand wholeness, to know that what occurs in one dimension of life affects all the others, and how to perceive problems in the dimensions outside of their discipline.
3. Training in team cooperation: such that physicians, staff, and spiritual caregivers can work together as a team, consulting with each other in order to move sick people toward healing and restoration of health
4. Dependence on God through prayer and regular consultation with him

The Problem of Modern Medicine

Medicine has multiple levels of trained personnel, from the auxiliary and technical levels through the highly specialized professional caregivers. The same multi-level approach to care for soul and spirit is important as well. In the area of psychology, we find middle level counselors and more highly trained psychologists and psychiatrists. What is lacking, however, is trained personnel on the primary level to provide care for the common and less complicated problems of mind, soul, and spirit that many sick persons have which may influence their physical health or recovery from illness. People with minor problems – loss of a loved one, a dysfunctional relationship, fear – do not always require the help of professional counselors. They may receive much benefit from a person trained to listen, to identify painful feelings of grief, fear, bitterness, or jealousy, and to provide simple counseling, encouragement, and spiritual care. Spiritual caregivers also need skills in identifying more complex problems that need referral to professional counseling staff. In this study, we call these primary level caregivers "spiritual caregivers." Others call them "helpers," or "lay ministers."

This study is intended for you who are being trained as a spiritual caregiver to be part of the healing team. We all need to understand wholeness from both spiritual and scientific perspectives, how to discover the whole story of a sick person, and how to work together with Christ as healer to bring healing and restoration to people.

In the current climate of multiculturalism, relativism, litigation, and often antagonism to the Christian faith, the question may arise: *Can this Christ-centered and spiritually oriented approach be done effectively and safely?* We believe it can if it is done with wisdom, much prayer, and avoidance of manipulation or coercion.

Medical care is now based on two important principles:
1. Patient-focused care
2. Scientific evidence that a certain therapy is beneficial

To these, we would add a third : Spiritual care

Patient-focused care
In this approach, we do nothing aside from that which a sick person wants done. We can offer prayer, but should never impose it. We can discuss spiritual issues only if the sick person so desires. Done with care and under the guidance of the Spirit of God, a Christ-centered approach to caring for the whole person is possible. This requires trained spiritual caregivers functioning alongside healthcare professionals in one setting. Many benefits will come both to sick persons receiving the care and to those providing the care.

Evidence-based care
Medicine does what we can prove scientifically to be effective. Medical science now has compelling evidence that psychosocial and spiritual factors in our lives affect us physically. Spirituality is "in," and can be discussed openly. Spiritual care has become "evidence-based care."

Spiritual care

Spiritual care is more than just talking to persons about Jesus and praying with them. It includes, but is not limited to, the following:

1. Inviting sick persons who are interested to come into a personal (covenant) relationship with God through Jesus Christ, or to renew or strengthen their relationship with him. Salvation is a process. It begins with conversion, then continues on through the rest of a person's life. It is salvation from:
   - the power of sin and temptation
   - thoughts, feelings, and attitudes contrary to God's revealed plan for our lives
   - all that would destroy our relationship with God.

2. Helping a person discover or recover a positive self-image. Many people suffer from low self-esteem. This may be caused by difficult life circumstances, an abusive family background, repeated failures, negative messages, etc. The message they need to understand is
   - God created them in his image.
   - God loves them.
   - God knows their name.
   - God has a good plan for their life.
   - God will work with them to discover that plan, as they are willing to let him.

3. Helping a person find something meaningful to do:
   - Finding a fulfilling job
   - Discovering one's creativity
   - Finding happiness on the various levels of life

4. Helping a person resolve inner conflicts, or finding healing for inner anguish or pain. Inner healing comes when we can bring our guilt, anger, grudges, bitterness, resentments, broken relationships, anxiety, worry, etc. to Jesus, release them to him and receive his provision of healing. Often this requires another wise person to help with this process. You may be that wise person who can help them.

5. Helping a person change thoughts or behavior patterns related to unhealthy attitudes or life style. This usually requires a long-term relationship with someone trained and experienced in this. The basic resource, however, is to come into a dynamic relationship with Jesus and realize that he has broken the power of destructive thoughts, behavior, or addictions that may be plaguing one's life.

6. Praying with all sick persons who want it: for healing, for resolution of personal problems, and for any other concerns. Always ask permission before praying. Once that is granted, a question such as: Are there other specific problems you would like me to pray about? This often uncovers other major concerns in the person's life that need to be dealt with.

Effective spiritual care within the medical environment has numerous important elements:

1. A team approach, in order to facilitate care for the whole person
   - physicians able to discern personal and spiritual concerns, usually by asking questions and truly hearing what a sick person says
   - trained spiritual caregivers who can minister to personal and spiritual issues as outlined above.
   - A sympathetic nursing and administrative staff

2. Long-term follow-up. Sick persons whom you care for spiritually should be encouraged to return at regular intervals for on-going support, evaluation of the current situation, and encouragement.

3. Awareness of community support structures to meet the basic needs of a sick person

4. Networking with spiritually alive churches or groups
   - for Bible study
   - spiritual growth
   - for opportunities to serve in the church and the community

From this it is clear that a community-based network that includes spiritually dynamic churches needs to be developed. This should be the goal of any Christian healthcare program that works to empower people spiritually, psychologically, and socially. Restoration to wholeness includes restoration to the community – family and other support groups – and the churches within the community should be prepared to respond and help.

Helping Hurting People

Questions for reflection
After reading this lesson, look at the questions below, reflect on them, and write in your answers in the space provided.

1. Make a list of what you feel are deficiencies in modern medicine in the areas of personal and psycho-spiritual care.

2. If you have been ill and received care, did those caring for you treat you as a person, or were they concerned simply for your physical, anatomical health? Did they inquire about your family, work, personal issues, or stress load? What do you wish they had done differently?

3. What suggestions can you make about how to improve modern healthcare?

Here is a situation to think about
Bill, while driving at 90 mph in his pick-up one night, crashed into a cement abutment. He was brought into the ER and found to have a fracture of the shaft of the femur, a lacerated liver, lung contusions, and internal head injuries. However, after expert medical and surgical care, he left the hospital six weeks later fully restored physically and could return to work.

1. Had he been restored to health as a whole person?

2. Is there more information you would like to have in order better to answer the first question? If so, ask your instructor about this.

Homework for lesson 2:
Read lesson two in *Helping Hurting People*.

Lesson 2
How Have We Gotten Into This Mess?

This lesson is optional. We will not spend much time on it in class. However, it helps us understand better where we are now if we know how we have gotten there. If you have questions about this, feel free to ask them.

The study of history can be very profitable. It helps us understand how we arrived at where we are now. It can also show us important lessons from the past, and, if we study them carefully, they can equip us to plan better for the future. To understand how medicine and healthcare have become so complex and deviated so far from the compassionate and self-sacrificing devotion of our forebears, we must go back into antiquity. Our brief study will involve philosophy and worldviews as well as history.

In ancient times, and in many cultures up until the present, illness is considered to be a spiritual and/or a social issue. Something has gone wrong in the life of a person. The Hebrews implicated sin against God and others as a major causal factor in illness. In the many forms of animistic cultures it is broken relationships with the gods, ancestral spirits, or with other people, and often involving a curse or evil eye. Among the ancient Greeks, it was imbalance in the forces of life. An understanding of physical causes of illness was minimal. Healing the sick took place in temples, and priests were not only mediators between people and the spiritual realm, but were also considered to be healers.

A fundamental question in philosophy is: How can we know truth? What are the ways we can discover truth? The two predominant philosophers among the Greeks, Plato and Aristotle, attempted to answer the 'truth' question. They both agreed that we can discover truth through sense observation and through reason, the intellectual evaluation of what the senses perceive. Plato believed we could find truth also in the spiritual realm, by studying Forms and finding basic principles of life. Aristotle objected to that. Forms may be real, he argued, but were personal, unreliable and arbitrary. We have no *proof* of their objective reality. Throughout the centuries prior to and just after Christ, the followers of Plato predominated in Greek thought, and this facilitated the spread of the Hebrew-Christian world view in the Hellenized and Roman worlds.

In Hebrew thought, revelation from God is the primary source of truth. Sense observation and reason are also valid because God, who is intelligent and perceptive, created us in his image with intellect and sense perception. We can discern truth through the study and analysis of nature because it has been created by God. What we find must then be submitted to what God himself has revealed about the nature of reality.

The remarkable compassionate care of the sick, widows, and orphans, and the philanthropy of the poor yet generous Christian community facilitated the rapid permeation of the Christian faith during the first three centuries of the Christian era. Hospices grew, and the care of sick persons whoever they were – slaves, wounded soldiers, and those suffering from "unclean" diseases – astounded the non-Christian world that tried without success to replicate this. This was especially evident in the widespread epidemics of small pox and other diseases during those early centuries. Compassionate care was the hallmark of the early Christian community. This declined markedly when the Christian faith became the official religion of the Roman Empire and the church became an institution of power, wealth, and authority. Spontaneous care of the sick now became the responsibility of monasteries and was institutionalized.

The conflict between the philosophies of Plato and Aristotle escalated during the first ten centuries of the Christian era, and gradually Aristotelian philosophy predominated. The Islamic civilization of the 8th through the 11th centuries reinforced Aristotelian philosophy and transferred it to Europe before Islamic culture began to decline. Aristotelian philosophy, or rationalism, which rejected the validity of revelation as a source of objective truth, threatened the church. St. Thomas of Aquinas attempted to reconcile the rationalism of Aristotle with the revelation found in the Bible. However, rationalism had a powerful appeal to the human ego for it made human wisdom the final court of appeal in deciding what is the truth. This eventually led to the Enlightenment that placed Man at the center of the universe.

The church finally had to incorporate rationalism in ecclesiastical philosophy. It did so quite adroitly by deciding that, in biblical times, God acted not only as creator but also as sustainer of the universe. In other words, God was imminent in creation as well as Lord of all creation. He acted in human history and miracles were frequent. However, now in post biblical times, God no longer acts in human history. Spiritual life is real, but is limited to our personal lives and eternal destiny. It has no practical implications. This effectively transferred God and the spiritual realm to "upstairs" – heaven, and to the future – eternal life after death. The culture of the West thus became a divided or split culture. God is; he enables us to find personal meaning and destiny, but the only sources of practical truth are what we perceive by our senses and intellect and what we can demonstrate by scientific validation. Matter and spirit are separate. Life is divided into the sacred (religious) which is personal and unverifiable, and the secular (practical life) which is our "real" or daily life. Healing still remained within the purview of the church.

This divided the Christian community. The orthodox churches embraced this philosophy. Other small groups – Anabaptists and pietists – rejected it and gave predominance to the imminence of God in daily life. Among those groups some, even until today, reject the scientific approach to health and healing and depend almost solely on prayer and faith.

Another major development in the philosophy of Christendom that has had a highly positive effect in western culture in general and medicine in particular was a deeper understanding of biblical values and their application to all of life. This came out of the Reformation which affirmed the importance of the individual person before God and in human life – "The just shall live by faith." The Reformation facilitated the translation of the Bible into many languages of the people. A deeper understanding of God's Word led to the "desacralization" of nature. Nature, and especially the human body, are not sacred and "off limits," but are valid subjects for study, analysis, and better understanding. This slowly liberated the scientific community and by the 17th century, significant advances occurred in our understanding of the natural world.

How Have We Gotten into This Mess?

As medical science advanced during the 18th and 19th centuries, the church realized that the ministry of healing now required those with special knowledge and training. This fit in with the already split world view of the West. Illness came to be recognized as primarily a disruption in the physical dimension of the person, so those trained in scientific analysis and treatment were best able to provide care. The church relegated to the medical community the care of the sick, retaining its care simply over the spiritual dimension of people. Eventually this separation became almost complete.

In the early 1900s a major controversy developed in the Johns Hopkins Faculty of Medicine between Sir William Osler, widely considered the 'father' of modern medicine, and Dr. William Welch, the dean of the medical school. It concerned the nature of medicine. For Osler, medicine is people, with the doctor/patient relationship being the primary concern. For Welch, medicine was science, and all else was secondary. Welch prevailed; Osler left, and medicine then veered sharply away from consideration of the person to verifiable scientific evidence. Tragically, neither of the men recognized that, in reality, these considerations are not polar opposites but are rather complementary, with both science and personal issues essential and compatible. The die was cast, however, and medicine became increasingly depersonalized.

The time-honored personal and family-oriented care of the "general practitioners" with their altruistic concern for people, gradually declined and almost disappeared. Practitioners became specialized, institutionalized, and increasingly technological. Without realizing it, health professionals themselves became depersonalized. The "caring physician" of yesterday has become the "bio-medical engineer" of today.

A second major controversy occurred at the Johns Hopkins School of Public Health in the 1970s over the nature of public health. Dr. Carl Taylor, professor of international health, argued that public health is horizontal, involving people and communities. Dr. Henderson, the dean, insisted that public health is vertical, top-down, and the purview of governments and legislation. Henderson prevailed, and in spite of an important effort by the World Health Organization at the Alma Ata international health conference in 1978 to make primary health care of the people predominant in government planning, public health has become vertical, institutionalized and extremely paternalistic.

In the meantime, as medical science made remarkable and beneficial advances, the ego of the medical community made greater advances, and a "Jehovah complex" developed among leaders of the medical community. Medical leadership assumed control of the decisions made about health care, and cut itself off from the community. The community lost ownership of health issues and could make little if any contribution to decisions about healthcare and facilities. Medical institutions became increasingly competitive, often to the detriment of the population who, in the final analysis, pay the bills. Health professionals, seeing the increasing revenues from medical care, quickly took advantage of this, and medicine became a highly remunerated profession at the expense of sick persons. Money and profit have become principal drivers in healthcare. Here is our picture of what our current healthcare system looks like:

STATE OF THE US HEALTHCARE SYSTEM

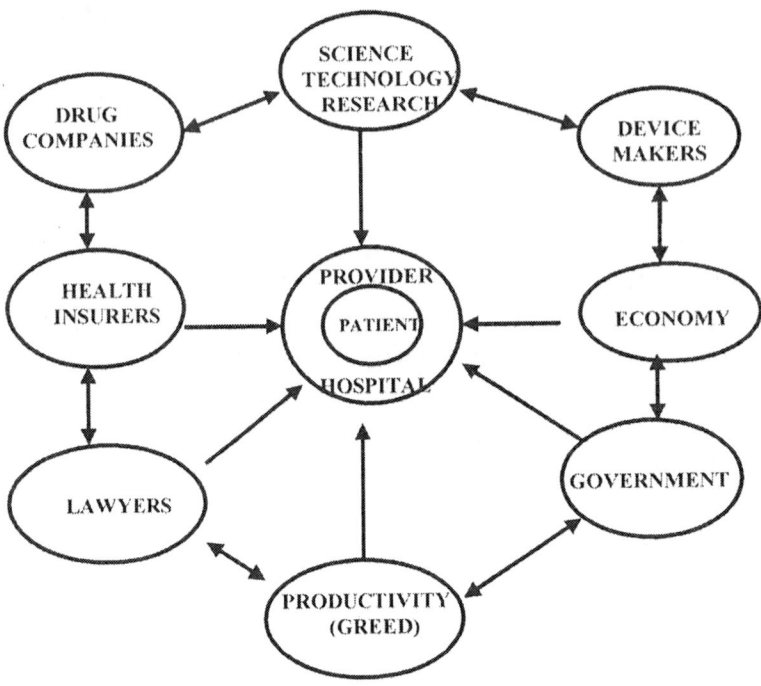

During the past century, churches have again realized they have a role in caring for the sick. Some churches engage in 'healing ministries,' with special services for prayer for healing. Active visitation of the sick in homes and hospitals is now widespread, with church leaders and members bringing comfort and encouragement to sick people. At the same time, the medical community increasingly recognizes that sick persons have 'religious needs' that should be met. Chaplaincy programs now exist in most major hospitals, and training programs in clinical pastoral education prepare church leaders for this specialized ministry. However, in many medical institutions, the pastoral care program is not well integrated into the life of the medical community, and chaplains and pastoral caregivers do their work separately from the medical and nursing staffs.

Within the past half century, decision-making power in healthcare has shifted markedly. No longer does the health profession have the final say, and sometimes has no say at all. Because of the almost total preoccupation with the physical aspects of diagnosis and treatment, the pharmaceutical industry has grown remarkably and is almost entirely commercialized and market oriented. Third-party payers, while necessary, have assumed major decision making roles, and the community is dealing with healthcare arrogance by having increasing recourse through the legal system.

Where do we go from here? Can this immense 'system' of the healthcare industry be changed? Some of us believe it can and desperately want to see that happen, but are deeply aware that outside interventions by government, legislation, or social forces can make little or no basic changes. Change must come from within. It must be 'horizontal,' not 'vertical'. And that involves us. However, it requires far more than simply adding prayer and Christian witness to the existing system. Trying to graft spiritual care onto an almost totally secular system is tenuous at best. Radical transformation is required. This will at best take many years and must involve a growing number of caregivers dedicated to the process.

How Have We Gotten into This Mess?

The fundamental change that must occur is at the very center of medicine: the sick person. We must restore wholeness to those for whom we care. This involves a **radical paradigm shift** on our part as health professionals – doctors, nurses, and all healthcare providers. It means a return to a biblically wholistic view of reality in which physical, psychological, relational, and spiritual dimensions of life are once again recognized as equally valid, completely integrated, and requiring care and consideration. In other words, we must restore wholeness to sick persons. We must bring God and personal faith back into the healing process, restore personal and family considerations to care, and rebuild relationships with the community at large and religious communities in particular. In the process, we ourselves will recover a sense of wholeness, of vocation, and of personal commitment to bringing the good news of health and healing to people and communities. Here is what we believe we must accomplish to restore wholeness to healthcare:

WHAT THE US HEALTHCARE SYSTEM SHOULD LOOK LIKE

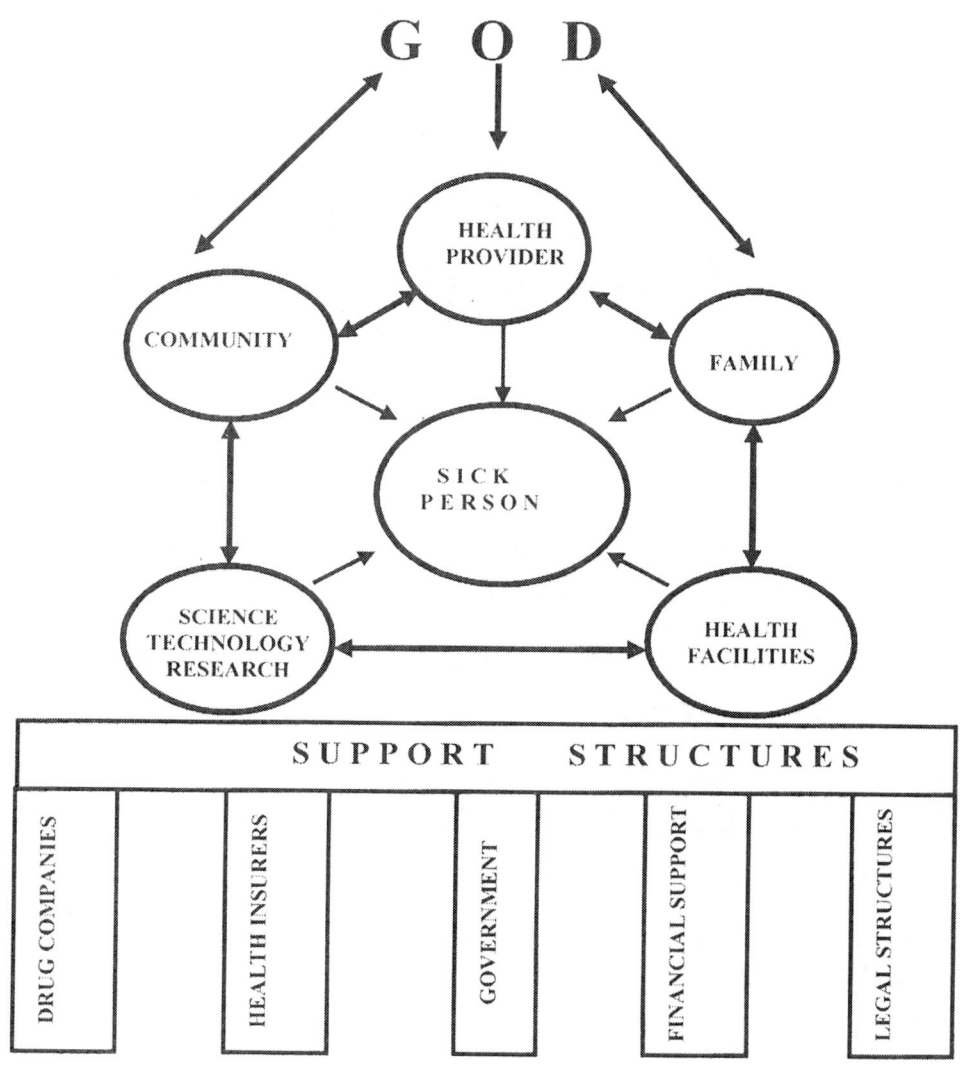

Helping Hurting People

Questions for reflection
1. List what you see as major philosophical developments and shifts, both positive and negative, that have occurred during the past 2500 years and now strongly influence the current healthcare system. (*Don't write a book! Just an outline.*)

2. What steps do you believe we, as trained and committed Christian caregivers, can take to restore compassionate care to medicine and bring faith and science, the church and medical care, back together?

Question for personal reflection
What role in the transformation of medicine as a healing ministry do you see yourself playing?

Bibliography:
Allen, Diogenes, *Christian Belief in a Postmodern World*, Westminster/John Know Press, Louisville, KY, 1989

Fountain, Daniel E., *Health, the Bible, and the Church*, Billy Graham Center, Wheaton, IL 1989

McGrath, Alister, *Bridge Building: Communicating Christianity Effectively*, IVP, 1992

Miller, Darrow, *Discipling the Nations*, YWAM, Seattle, 1998. A study of world views and how an understanding of them is helpful in transmitting the gospel.

Moreau, Scott, *A Sure Foundation*, unpublished, The Summer Medical Institute, 3512 Tilden St., Philadelphia, PA 19129 www.pediatricstoday.com/smi

Stark, Rodney, *The Rise of Christianity*, Harper, San Francisco 1997 – How the obscure marginal Jesus Movement became the dominant religious force in the western world in a few centuries.

In preparation for the next session, read chapter 2 in *God, Medicine, and Miracles* and lesson 3 in *Helping Hurting People*

Lesson 3
Jesus as our Model
Read also: God, Medicine, and Miracles, *chapter two*

Compassionate care for sick persons as whole persons, whoever they are, began with Jesus. Jesus did indeed cure diseases such as leprosy, convulsive disorders, and physical handicaps; however, he went much beyond the physical healings to restore people to <u>wholeness.</u>

The Hebrew word from which the name Jesus comes is *Yeshuwah*. It means "to save, to heal, to restore, to make whole." So the name *Jesus* means all of these things. Let's look at an example of how he saved, healed, and restored a sick woman.

A 'case study'
In Mark's Gospel, chapter 5, verses 25 - 34, is the account of how Jesus healed a woman with a serious gynecological problem. This is how Mark reports this 'case study.'

There was a woman who had suffered terribly from severe bleeding for twelve years, even though she had been treated by many doctors. She had spent all her money, but instead of getting better she got worse all the time. She had heard about Jesus, so she came in the crowd behind him, saying to herself, "If I just touch his clothes, I will get well." She touched his cloak, and her bleeding stopped at once; and she had the feeling inside herself that she was healed of her trouble. At once Jesus knew that power had gone out of him, so he turned around in the crowd and asked, "Who touched my clothes?" His disciples answered, "You see how the people are crowding you; why do you ask who touched you?" But Jesus kept looking around to see who had done it. The woman realized what had happened to her, so she came, trembling with fear, knelt at his feet, and told him the whole truth. Jesus said to her, "My daughter, your faith has made you well. Go in peace, and be healed of your trouble."

As we examine stories in the Bible like this, it is helpful to use our imagination and add to the account details that most certainly were present yet not recorded. We need the help of God's Spirit to do this, as prayerful and careful analysis of details not recorded in the text can help us better grasp the whole story. We will do that here.

Stop here and take a few minutes to analyze this story.

List the physical symptoms, social issues, and psycho-spiritual problems this woman probably had but that were not recorded by Mark. Use your imagination to fill out the details of this story. Take a separate sheet of paper and make an enlarged table like this:

	Problems of the woman	How Jesus healed them
Physical		
Social		
Psycho-spiritual		

How did Jesus heal her in all these areas of her life?

This woman had a gynecological problem - severe bleeding for twelve years. Mark does not give us the diagnosis (he was not a physician). It surely was not cancer, or another type of tumor, for the history is too long and Jewish women rarely got cancer of the uterus. Most likely it was a hormonal imbalance. With this history of bleeding, she surely was anemic from the chronic loss of blood, and therefore tired and weak, thus being unable to fulfill her duties as a woman. She probably had no children, for at least during this 12 year period, she had been unable to conceive.

She likewise had serious social problems. As a Jew, she was constrained by the Old Testament Law, and in the book of Leviticus (chapter 15) we find detailed laws concerning bleeding, how it renders a person unclean, and what must be done to become clean again. Not only was this woman continuously unclean, but everything and everyone she touched became unclean. She was socially ostracized for twelve years - a frightful burden for anyone. If she had once been married, her husband had abandoned her. Even family and friends could not accept her, visit her, or allow her to come to their homes for she would render them unclean. Also, she was penniless, as Mark mentions in the text.

Imagine, therefore, what feelings were in this woman's heart - a sense of rejection, grief, and probably anger directed against society and even against God who had allowed this tragedy to come to her. Finally, spiritually she was cut off even from God himself, for no unclean person could go to the Temple to pray, confess sins, offer a gift, or ask for help. So what Mark reports here is not just a 'gynecological case.' He states clearly: 'There was a <u>woman</u> who suffered terribly,' in the totality of her life.

She then heard about Jesus, an important man who could heal those who were ill. She desperately wanted to go to him, but she could not, for she would make him unclean. Therefore she came up with a dangerous plan - to sneak up behind him in a crowd and simply touch the tassel on his robe, even though it would make Jesus unclean. It was crucial that no one see her do this because, were she detected, the Jewish culture required that she be severely censured and perhaps even stoned. Yet, because of her condition, she had nothing to lose, so she went ahead and accomplished her plan.

Her faith was rewarded, for instantly she felt the bleeding drying up within her. She knew she then had to escape immediately. But it was Jesus himself who stopped her and exposed her publicly. Why did Jesus do that? He knew she had been healed physically. Why was he not content with that? As a physician, I have cared for thousands of women with problems similar to those of this woman. When I (DF) was able to cure their bleeding, or their infertility, I was happy and so were they. Why was Jesus not satisfied? It was simply because the <u>woman herself</u> had not yet been healed.

When the woman came back to Jesus she was frightened to death, for she knew what she had done. She had made this important man unclean. Even worse, she had stolen his power. She was sure, therefore, she was going to be condemned. However, as she lay at Jesus' feet, instead of a word of condemnation, she heard an incredible word, just one word, a word that healed her in the totality of her being. She heard Jesus call her his daughter. At that moment, all of the rejection, loss of self-esteem, grief, and anger melted away, and in the depths of her heart she was healed. Jesus then lifted her up and made restoration to her family and community possible. The word Jesus spoke set her free!

Medicine has many interventions for healing the body. But what heals the broken heart and the wounded spirit of a person? What can take away the anguish, pain, guilt, or conflicts in the heart? Remarkably, it is very simple. It is simply a WORD that heals the heart. The Bible calls it a '*rhema*' word. It is not just any word, however. Rather it is the specific word the heart longs to hear that speaks to the anguish, the conflicts, and the pain and resolves them. (Proverbs 25:11)

How did Jesus heal this woman?
1. <u>He used physical power</u> to heal the bleeding. We do not have his miraculous power, but we do have physical power to heal. By the wisdom God has given us, we have developed other types of power - medicines, surgery, and a broad spectrum of technology that we can, in full faith, use for physical healing.

2. <u>He listened to her story</u>, the whole story. Hurting people are usually desperate to have someone who will truly listen to them. Here, however, is our problem. We do not take the time to listen to the stories of hurting people, and every one has a story. So we do not know the burdens they are carrying. It is helpful to remember where Jesus was when the woman told him her story. He was rushing to Jairus' house because Jairus' daughter was dying. Yet he took the time to listen to this woman. Here is where trained spiritual caregivers fit in, for they will have the time to listen to hurting people.
3. In listening to her story, <u>Jesus discerned her real problem</u> - rejection, anger against God, and total abandonment. We need to ask God to give us real discernment of inner problems as we listen to hurting persons.
4. <u>Jesus then knew the word her heart needed to hear,</u> a word of acceptance and of restoration of dignity. In this case, that single word "my daughter" was all she needed for the healing of her broken heart and wounded spirit. Often, when we discern the underlying problem(s), we can then know the healing word the heart of the person needs to hear.
5. He made <u>restoration</u> to her family and community possible.

These last four are the interventions that spiritual caregivers will learn to make. Added to medical knowledge, skills, and technology, all of this can bring help, even healing, to the whole person. Now let's look more closely at the healing power of a word or message spoken to the heart.

<u>Words that heal</u>
Psychology shows us clearly the immense distance between the mind – our thoughts – and the heart – our feelings. What we see and hear, and the thoughts that come from this, often do not penetrate into the feelings of the heart *because they do not fit*. Our reason tells us one thing; our heart feels the opposite. For example, I may KNOW in my mind that God has forgiven me, but I FEEL in my heart that God cannot forgive me. We need to understand this, because the key to healing the broken heart is *finding the words that fit what the heart needs to hear*. Here is how it works:

1. The mind (intellect, reason) deals with thoughts. Thoughts come from the words we hear, the things we see, touch, taste, or feel.
2. The heart takes these thoughts, gives them an emotional content, and interprets them.
3. The emotional interpretation is far more powerful and more deeply retained than is the mental image (thoughts).
4. The inner pain, anxiety, anguish people feel is in their hearts, in their emotions, and in their feelings. For healing of this inner pain, the <u>heart</u> must hear a word that speaks to that pain. The heart must accept it and recognize that this word has resolved the tension, conflict, and pain.
5. On the other hand, if the emotional interpretation of a thought or word does not 'fit' the feelings in the heart, it is rejected. It "goes in one ear and out the other."
6. The challenge, as helpers, is to hear the <u>Rhema Word</u> the heart of a person needs to hear, the word that *fits* the emotional pain and resolves it.

In the book of Isaiah we find a remarkable passage that describes this. God is calling Isaiah to go and speak to the people of Israel, but he warns Isaiah that they are a stubborn people. He tells him:

Jesus as Our Model

Go and tell this people: "Be ever hearing, but never understanding;
be ever seeing, but never perceiving.
You will be ever hearing, but never understanding;
You will be ever seeing, but never perceiving.
Otherwise, you might see with your eyes, hear with your ears,
Understand with your hearts, and turn and be healed." (Isaiah 6: 9 – 10)

This shows very clearly the 'route' for healing the broken heart:
1. Thoughts in the mind come from what is seen or heard.
2. The interpretation and understanding of these thoughts takes place in the heart.
3. When the heart accepts the understood message, this allows that word to resolve the pain and anguish of the heart.

Reflect on this story
1. What did the <u>heart</u> of the woman with bleeding hear Jesus say that healed her inner pain?
2. How did that single word resolve the long-standing anguish of her heart?
3. What kind of words speak to the depths of the heart?

Look at the story of Deborah, a Jewish woman, divorced, in despair, and suicidal, as it is told in *GMM*, pages 49 and 50. Discuss together what Deborah's real problems were.
- How did Jesus heal her broken heart?
- Do you know someone with a problem like Deborah's?
- How could you help that person?

Analyze the story of John, dying of tuberculosis in spite of adequate medical treatment – see *GMM* pages 35-38.

1. What were the real problems in his heart?

2. What healing words did his heart hear and understand?

3. How did the words heal him and restore him to wholeness?

The following diagrams may help you:

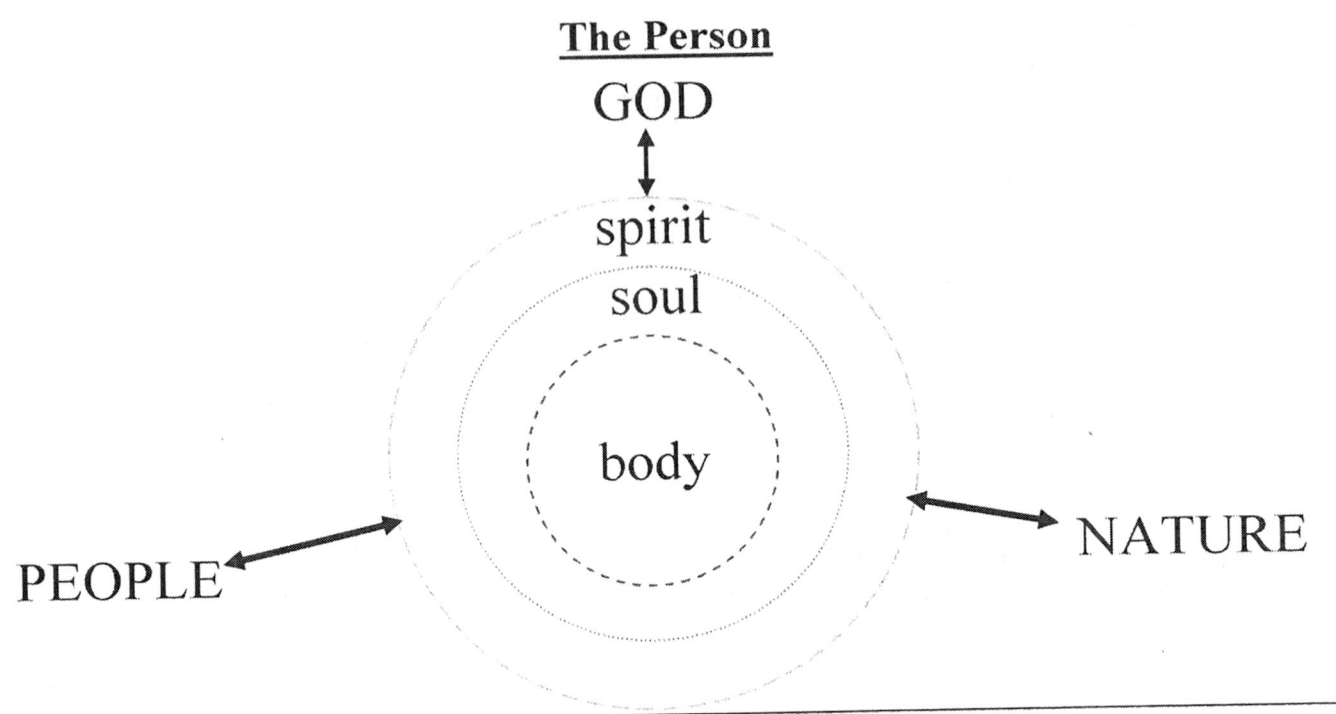

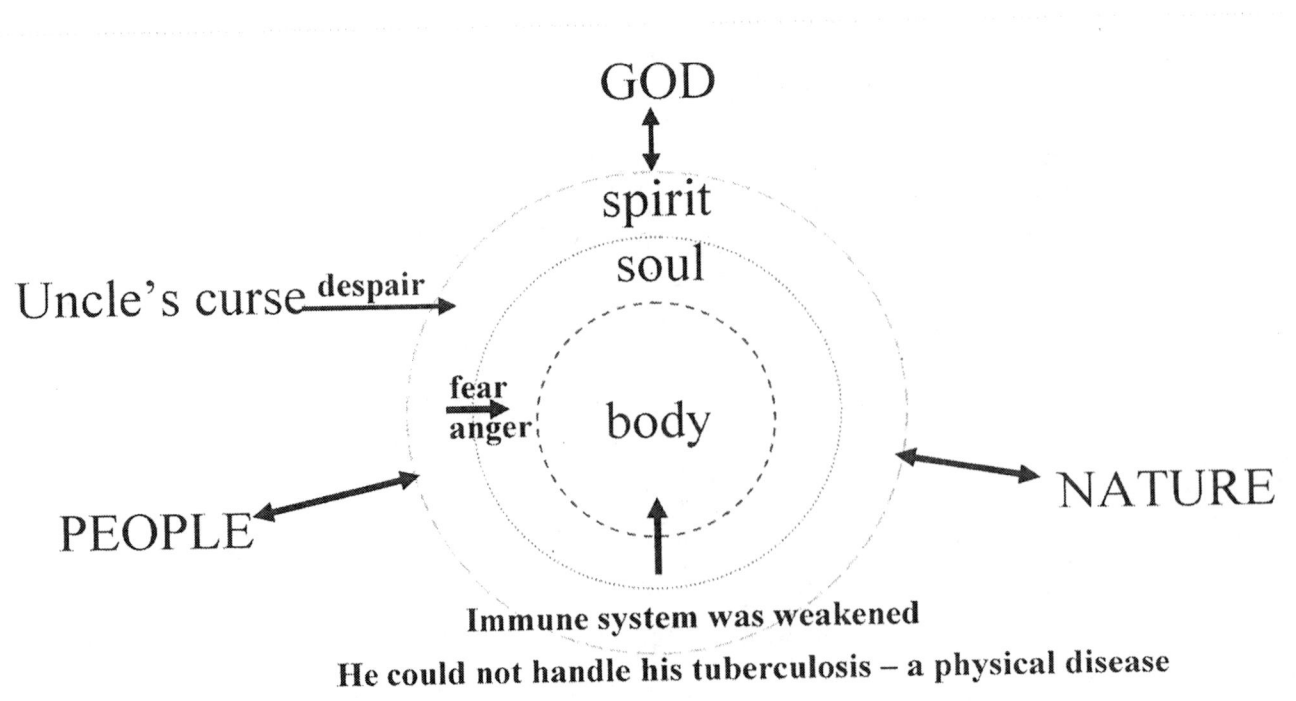

Jesus as Our Model

HOW JESUS HEALED JOHN'S PROBLEMS

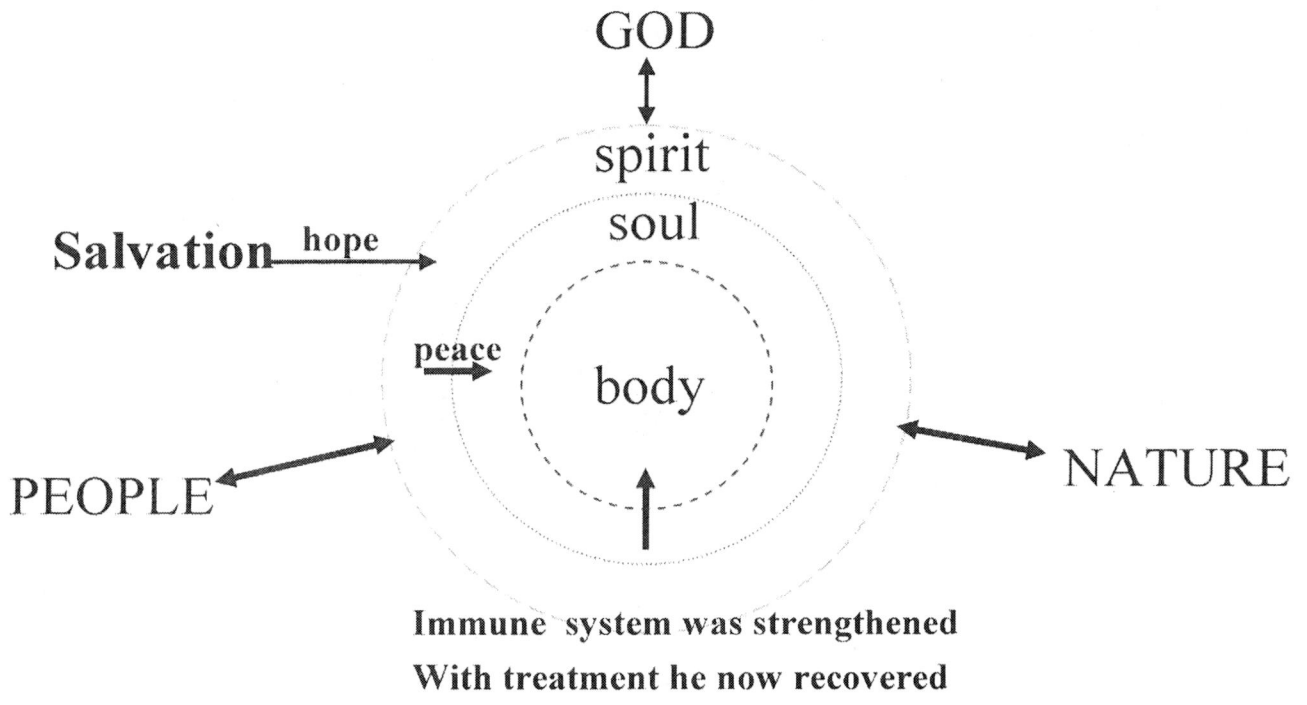

**Immune system was strengthened
With treatment he now recovered**

Consider these questions

1. Why is there such a great 'distance' between the head and the heart?

2. Have you ever had a healing word spoken to you? Or to someone in your family? Describe it here

3. Have you ever had harmful words spoken to you that have brought grief or anguish? Describe one such harmful word here. What did it do to you?

Optional but instructive further study

Look at the following examples of Jesus' healing ministry to see how he cared for the whole person. Answer these questions for each one:

a. How did the illness affect the person physically, psychologically, spiritually, and in social relationships?

b. How did Jesus bring healing in each of the dimensions of the sick person's life?
- The man with leprosy – Mark 1 : 40 – 45
- The paralyzed man - Mark 2 : 1 – 12
- The man with the withered hand – Mark 3 : 1-6; cf Luke 6 : 6 – 11
- The man with an evil spirit – Mark 1 : 21 – 27
- The man who was blind and dumb – Matthew 12 : 22 – 32
- The daughter of Jairus – Mark 5 : 21 – 43
- The man with many evil spirits – Mark 5 : 1 – 20
- The man born blind – John 9 : 1 – 34

What can we conclude from these studies about how Jesus healed sick people?

What does this teach us about how we are to heal people today?

Additional reading

The following book provides narrative accounts of most of these healings:
Who Is This Man Jesus? - Dan Fountain, Selah Books, 2003 – www.selahbooks.com or www.amazon.com

Homework
1. Read chapter 3 in *God, Medicine, and Miracles*
2. Read lesson 4 in *Helping Hurting People*

Lesson 4
The Biblical Perspective on Wholeness
Read also: God, Medicine, and Miracles, *chapter three*

This lesson is very important. We need to know what God says about both health and healing, and what God's will is considering our health. Does he want us to be healthy? We know that many diseases exist and that we are all susceptible to them. Are they part of God's plan for us? What does the Bible say about this?

There are several biblical teachings that make it clear that God's primary will for us is health. We will outline them briefly here, but we encourage you to study this further on your own.

1. In the Garden of Eden, disease, suffering, and death were not present because they were not part of God's primary plan for human life.
2. Disease and death came into human history when our first ancestors rebelled against the will of God. They chose disorder over the marvelous order God had created. So disease and death are in the world because of human disobedience, not because of the will of God.
3. God gave us many laws about health, with the clear teaching that if we obey those laws, this will favor our health, for example Deuteronomy 28 : 1 – 14. We find some of these laws in the Bible. We find many others that God has built into nature and into our bodies through the discoveries of science. If it is God's will for us to be sick at times, why did he give us so many laws that favor health?
4. His Son Jesus came to do his Father's will. Jesus healed sick people. From this it is clear that God not only wills our health but wants to heal us when we are sick. He even calls himself *Jehovah Rapha*, the God who heals us (Exodus 15 : 26).
5. God built marvelous mechanisms into our bodies to protect us from many diseases. We call this our *immune system* and we will study this in lesson 5. This is further evidence that God wants us to be healthy.
6. Finally, in eternity there is no disease, degeneration, disorder, or death. These are not part of God's eternal plan for us.

We can conclude from this that, as we make efforts to help sick people recover their health, we are working within God's will. If we consult God regularly as we do this, he will give us wisdom through his Word and his Spirit. We may even see occasions where God acts directly to heal someone. If this is so, why are so many people not healed in spite of our immense efforts and much prayer? Let's leave that difficult question until a few lessons later.

Let's now look at the biblical basis for knowing that we are whole persons because God made us that way. We are not composed of separate unrelated parts that God has somehow stuck together. Rather we are <u>one person</u>, with different aspects that are all intimately related to and influence each other. Let's look at key passages that describe our wholeness.

And God said, "Let us make man in our image, in our likeness, and let them rule over the fish of the sea and the birds of the air, over the livestock, over all the earth, and over all the creatures than move along the ground." So God created man in his own image, in the image of God he created him. Male and female he created them (Genesis 1: 26 -28 NIV).

Stop here and think about what this teaches us about ourselves.
1. List the many characteristics of God that he has put within us (his image).
2. What does this say about gender relationships?

Consider this passage:

> The Lord God formed the man from the dust of the ground and breathed into his nostrils the breath of life, and man became a living being. (Genesis 2: 7 NIV)

List some of the many wonderful physical organs God made out of dust. Start with the skin and work your way back inside the body.
1. How did he fit them all together?
2. How long do you suppose it took God to design all these organs and fit them together in such an intricate way that they can function harmoniously?
3. Consider the brain with its 26 billions neurons, each with 100 connections to other neurons. How do you suppose God designed that circuitry?
4. When God had completed the human body, was it alive?
5. What did God have to put into the body to make it alive?
6. So as whole persons, what are we made of?
7. Compare how God made us with how he made the animals – Gen. 2:19. What difference do you see in the way God made Man and the way he made animals?

Now listen to Jesus.

> Jesus answered, "Love the Lord your God with all your <u>heart,</u> with all your <u>soul</u>, with all your <u>mind,</u> and with all your <u>strength (body</u>). This is the greatest and the most important commandment. The second most important commandment is like it: Love your neighbor as you love yourself." (Matthew 22: 37 – 39)

1. What does this statement tell us about who we are as persons?
2. What are essential aspects of our life?
3. How do these aspects affect our health?

Let's look at Jesus himself in Luke 2: 52. How was he a whole person?

> Jesus grew both in <u>body</u> and in <u>wisdom</u>, gaining favor with <u>God</u> and <u>men</u>.

He grew in body, in mind (intellect and reason), in spirit (in his walk with God) and in relationships with other people. He was a whole person, and so are we.

The Biblical Perspective on Wholeness

Here is another key verse:

> May the God who gives us peace make you holy in every way and keep your whole being – spirit, soul, and body – free from every fault at the coming of our Lord Jesus Christ. (I Thessalonians 5:23)

What does this verse tell us about ourselves? How are we 'triune' beings?

Look now at a verse that describes a fundamental principle about human life, a principle that has great medical and psychological importance for us:

> Peace of mind makes the body healthy; but jealousy is like a cancer.
> (Proverbs 14: 30)

What does this verse say about the relationship between the mind (heart) and the body? Which one rules over the other?

Here is another important passage:

> And (Jesus) went on to say, "It is what comes out of a person that makes him unclean. For from the inside, from a person's heart, come the evil ideas which lead him to do immoral things, to rob, kill, commit adultery, be greedy, and do all sorts of evil things; deceit, indecency, jealousy, slander, pride, and folly – all these evil things come from inside a person and make him unclean."
> (Mark 7: 20-23)

The word 'unclean' can also mean 'sick.' How can these thoughts, feelings, and emotions make us sick, not only emotionally but physically as well? We will look at this in detail in the lessons that follow.

<u>Frequently used words</u>
   Before we continue, we need to clarify the meaning we are giving here to certain key words. These are not *definitions* because these concepts are too broad to be constrained by a strict definition. However, we do need a common understanding of what we mean by each of the words.

<u>Mind</u>: Thoughts, intellect, reason

<u>Soul</u>: Feelings, emotions, beliefs, memories, desires

<u>Spirit</u>: Our inmost being :
  - Where we are in contact with God, or other spiritual powers
  - Where we ask the basic questions of life: Who am I? Why am I alive? Where am I going? How am I supposed to live?
  - The seat of our will – where we make basic decisions about self and about life.

Heart: The Bible uses the word 'heart' to include mind, soul, and spirit. It is another way of stating 'our inner being."

Psyche: This is a more scientific term for mind and soul

Other important words
  We must distinguish between disease and illness, and between curing and healing.

Disease: A *particular condition* that upsets the normal functioning of a person.
  It can come from the outside – flu, pneumonia, an accident, etc.
  It can come from changes inside – high blood pressure, diabetes, etc.

Illness *has to do with the person.* It is all the uncomfortable feelings that come when a disease is present.

Curing has to do with disease. It means getting rid of the disease. Some diseases we can cure; others we cannot.

Healing has to do with the person. It is restoring the person to health. Healing of mind, soul, and spirit are almost always possible even if a cure is not possible.

The spiritual factor in healing – Faith

This involves four important elements:

1. The active power of God to heal.

2. The faith of sick persons that God can heal them. This is what brings them to God for healing. Their own faith may be strong or weak, clear, vague, or even absent. Our faith does not heal us. God heals us when **in faith** we go to him and ask him for healing.

3. The faith of family and friends. This operates through prayer, encouragement, and tender loving care. They can help sick persons bring the healing power of God into the caring relationship.

4. The faith of us who are giving care. Our faith in Jesus' power to resolve inner problems and thus to bring new strength to the body is what motivates us to bring people to Jesus for healing. Note the remarkable statement in Luke 2:5 – "Seeing how much faith **they had**, Jesus said to the sick man…."

The Biblical Perspective on Wholeness

Questions for reflection

1. Describe God's will concerning our health, and give biblical references for it.

2. What would you say to a person who believes his or her illness is the 'will of God'?

3. Document, with biblical references, what the Bible teaches about our **wholeness** as human beings?

4. How can we apply these teachings to helping hurting people?

Questions for your personal reflection

Are your own relationships with God, others, and yourself such as to reinforce your health, or perhaps to weaken it?

To whom could you go for help in resolving inner problems?

Homework
1. Read chapter 4 in *God, Medicine, and Miracles*
2. Read lesson 5 in *Helping Hurting People*

Lesson 5
The Heart/Body Relationship from the Scientific Perspective
God, Medicine, and Miracles, *Chapter four*

Medical science is discovering more and more evidence of how thoughts, feelings, emotions, desires, and even spirituality affect the organs of our body. How do you feel physically when you are afraid? Or when you are angry? Or when you are sad and upset?

For example, someone suddenly shouts "FIRE!" and you see smoke coming under the door. What happens to your heart rate? Your blood pressure? Your muscles?

When you are going through a time of intense stress or conflict, how well do you eat? Or sleep? Do you get symptoms like diarrhea, itching, or pains in various places?

We have all heard stories of someone displaying superhuman strength or speed when faced with a life-threatening situation or when trying to snatch a loved one from danger. Such stories demonstrate the amazing 'fight-or-flight' response of the physical body to the intense emotions of anger or fear.

All of these are normal physical responses that enable us to protect ourselves and do what needs to be done to cope with the acute problem. What is <u>not normal</u>, however, is to hold onto fear, anger, or jealousy for months or even years because, over time, this can make us physically ill.

How do thoughts, feelings, and emotions affect the functioning of our physical organs? Basically, our physical body responds to our thoughts and feelings through our hormones and through the brain.

<u>Hormones</u>
Glands like the adrenal glands produce chemicals called hormones in response to our thoughts and feelings. These hormones enter the blood stream immediately, circulate throughout the entire body, and influence all of our organ systems. When the fire alarm goes off, your adrenal glands instantly produce a large amount of <u>adrenalin</u>. The adrenalin immediately acts on your heart to increase its rate and pressure It also acts on your muscles to increase their blood supply and strength to enable you to run or do whatever else you need to do in this emergency.

The feelings resulting from stress also stimulate the adrenal gland to produce an increased quantity of <u>cortisol,</u> a hormone that enables the body to develop a defense to the spread of bacteria through wounds. We call this an inflammatory reaction; it defends us from widespread infections. These hormones, and others as well, affect the physical functioning of our organs to enable us to cope with the stresses of life.

<u>The brain</u>
The brain is our communication and control center. What we perceive by our senses comes into the brain through the nerves from our sense organs. The brain is linked to every organ and tissue in our body. Nerves from the brain carry electrical impulses to the organs and from the organs back to the brain. Our perceptions of the world around us are directly linked, therefore, with all of our physical organs.

Brain cells also manufacture chemicals called <u>neurochemicals</u>. The brain cells put these chemicals directly into the blood stream and they are carried immediately throughout the body in the circulation. These chemicals act on our organs and tissues.

Brain cells make neurochemicals in response to our emotions. For each emotion a particular neurochemical is made which has a specific action on our various organs. Positive emotions stimulate the production of neurochemicals that strengthen the functioning of our organs. Joy, peace, tranquility, and pleasure help our organs function harmoniously.

"Negative" emotions, such as shame, guilt, envy, lust, etc., stimulate the brain to produce neurochemicals that, over time, can have deleterious effects on our health:
- high blood pressure
- over-secretion of gastric acid, or spasms in the intestines
- inflammatory reactions in various tissues and organs
- chronic headaches and pain from tense muscles
- weakness, fatigue

Just as intense emotions such as fear or anger stimulate the adrenal glands to produce adrenalin, so they also cause the brain to produce neurochemicals that prepare the body for immediate action. They act on all of our various organs to keep them in a state of readiness to protect ourselves. The short term effects are not harmful to health. If we hold onto these intense 'defensive' feelings, however, the long term effects can be detrimental, for they cause our organs to maintain an unnecessary state of readiness.

From this we see the truth in Proverbs 14:30: "Peace of mind makes the body healthy; but jealousy is like a cancer." We know that cancer destroys the body. So also can envy, jealousy, suppressed anger, fear, and so on. Helping people find healing for these negative emotions is a principal objective of this helping ministry.

The immune system

God has created within us a system of defense against infections and certain malignancies. We call this the immune system. The immune system is made up of white blood cells, antibodies, and other products that circulate in the blood and the tissues to fight against these diseases. When an infection occurs, the body produces more white blood cells and antibodies. If the immune system is weak, it cannot produce enough white blood cells, and the body cannot resist the infection effectively.

We have numerous types of white blood cells:
1. CD_4 cells are like police. They identify invading organisms and give orders to other cells to attack them.
2. Phagocytes. They attack bacteria directly, eat them up, and destroy them.
3. Lymphocytes. Many of these produce antibodies (poisons) against the invading organisms.
4. Killer cells. These cells identify abnormal cancer-producing cells and destroy them.

We can strengthen our own immune system by paying attention to certain important measures:
1. Good food – eating a balanced diet
2. Plenty of stimulating exercise

The Heart/Body Relationship from the Scientific Perspective

3. Adequate rest and sleep
4. Protecting ourselves from infectious diseases
5. Inner healing and maintaining a sense of peace and joy in our hearts.

Our thoughts, feelings and emotions affect the immune system, namely our white blood cells and antibodies. Good feelings, like joy and peace, increase the production of white blood cells and antibodies and therefore increase our resistance to infections and our ability to fight against infections and malignancies. On the other hand, long-lasting painful feelings and destructive emotions like fear, anger, and envy diminish the production of white blood cells and antibodies. We then become more susceptible to colds, the flu, and other infections and less able to protect ourselves from them.

Think back to the story of John who had tuberculosis (*GMM pages 35-38*). In view of what we have just described, explain:
1. Why the medical treatment by itself did not work
2. Why his immune system was unable to fight against the tuberculosis germs
3. What happened to his soul and spirit to restore his immune system to normal
4. How the staff cared for him *as a whole person*
5. The final result and how it came about

We can picture this as a simple balance scale, with a weighing pan on each side. When a person becomes ill, it is as if the immune system is on one weighing pan and the disease on the other. The outcome of an infection and even some malignancies depends on the relative strength of the disease and the immune system. A strong healthy immune system can usually cope successfully with a major infection and even fight effectively against cancer. However, an immune system weakened by poor nutrition, worry, depression, or other negative emotions cannot respond adequately to such problems.

An infection has come. The outcome depends on which is stronger (or heavier) - the infection, or the immune system.

The disease/immune system balance

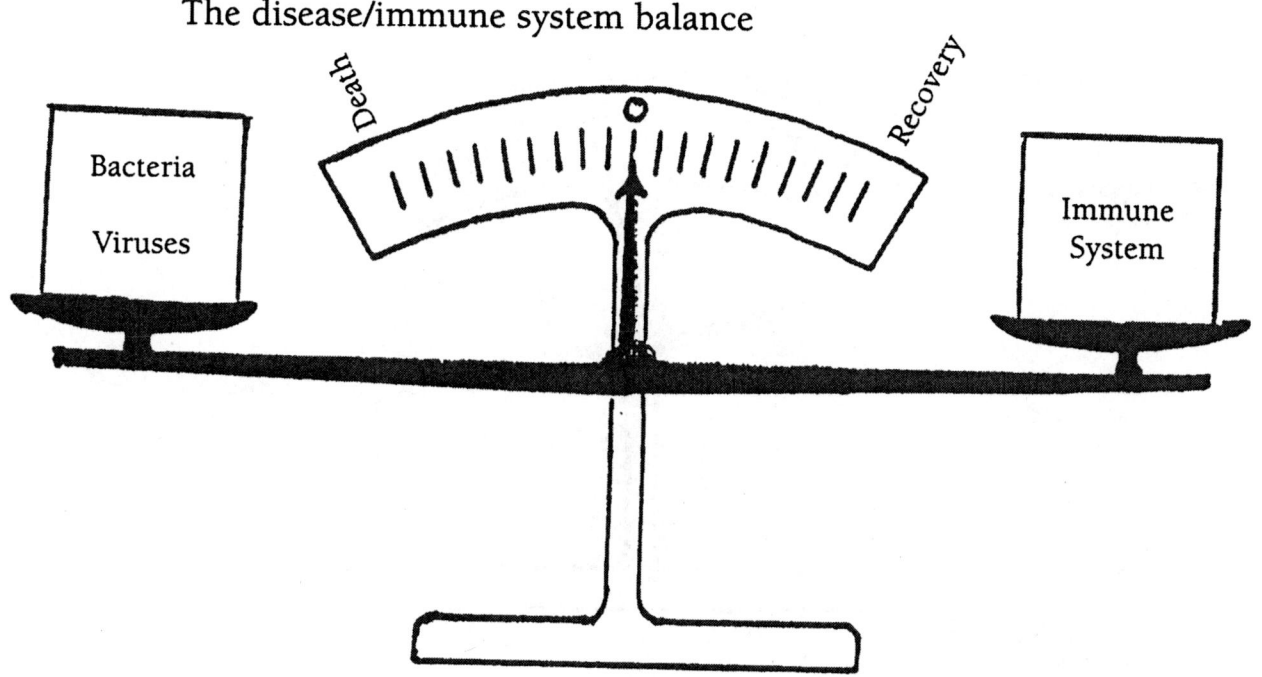

Poor food, fatigue, and stress weaken the immune system and the infection gets worse.

A weakened immune system

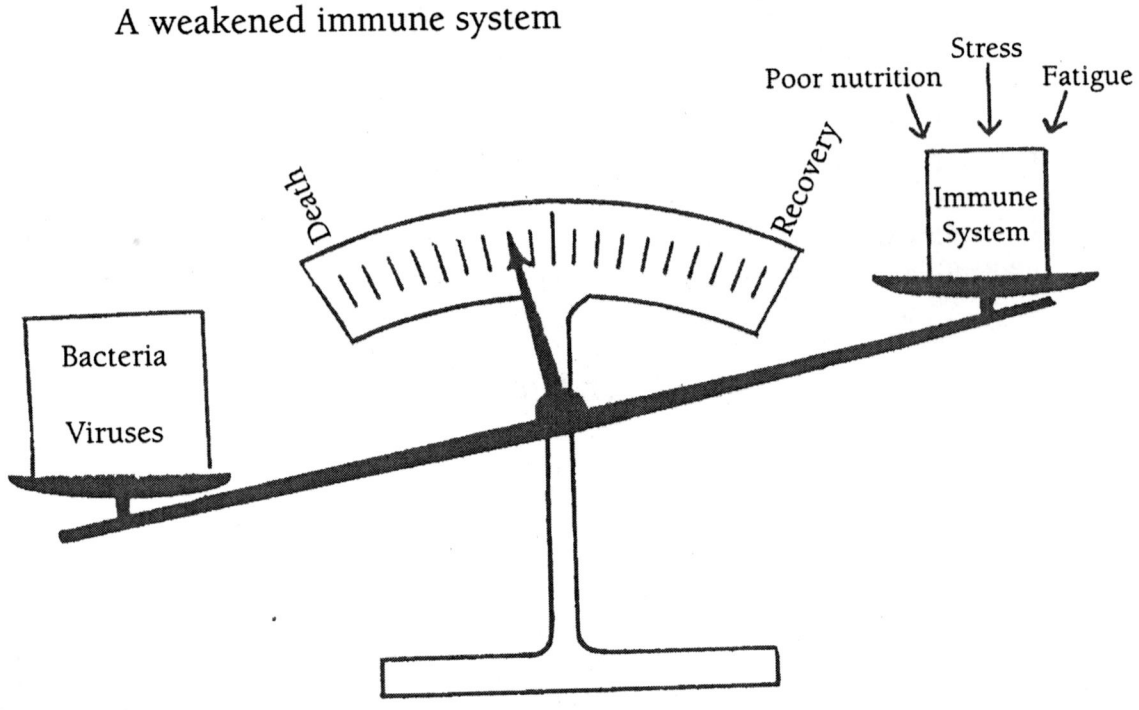

Antibiotics attack the disease organisms causing the infection. Good medical care helps the immune system to overcome the infection. The person can now get well.

Medical care and the fight against disease

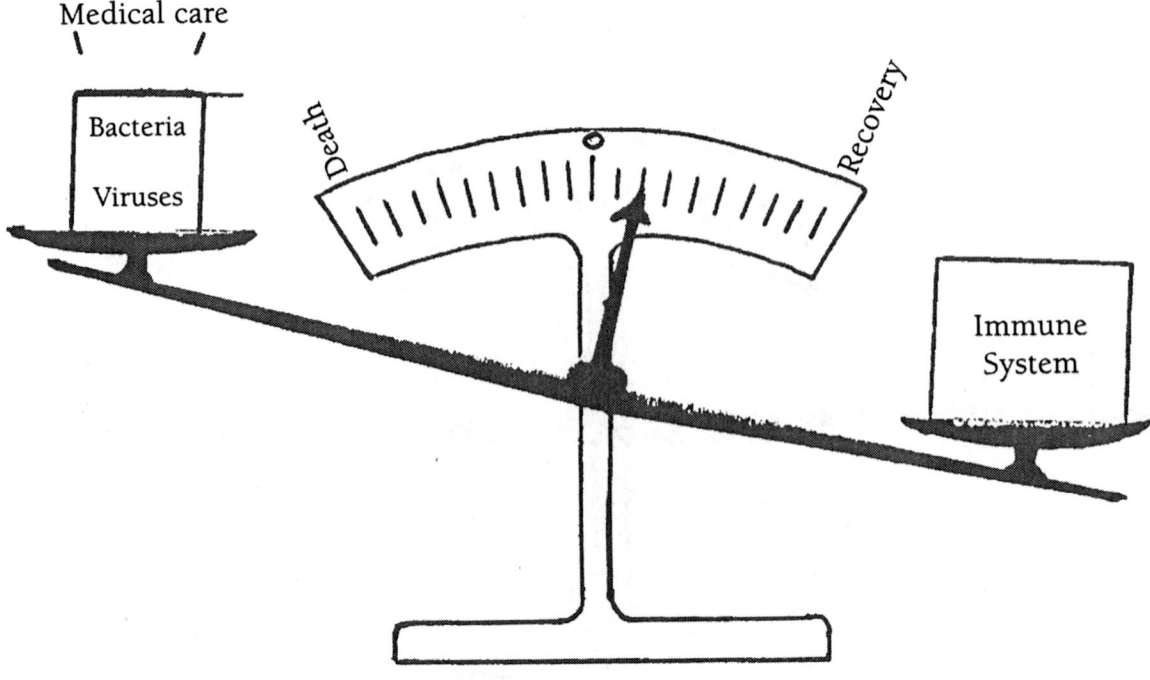

The Heart/Body Relationship from the Scientific Perspective

If we can help a sick person to get rid of negative emotions and find peace of mind, this will help his immune system become stronger. The immune system can now overcome the infection and the person can get well.

Peace of mind and the immune system

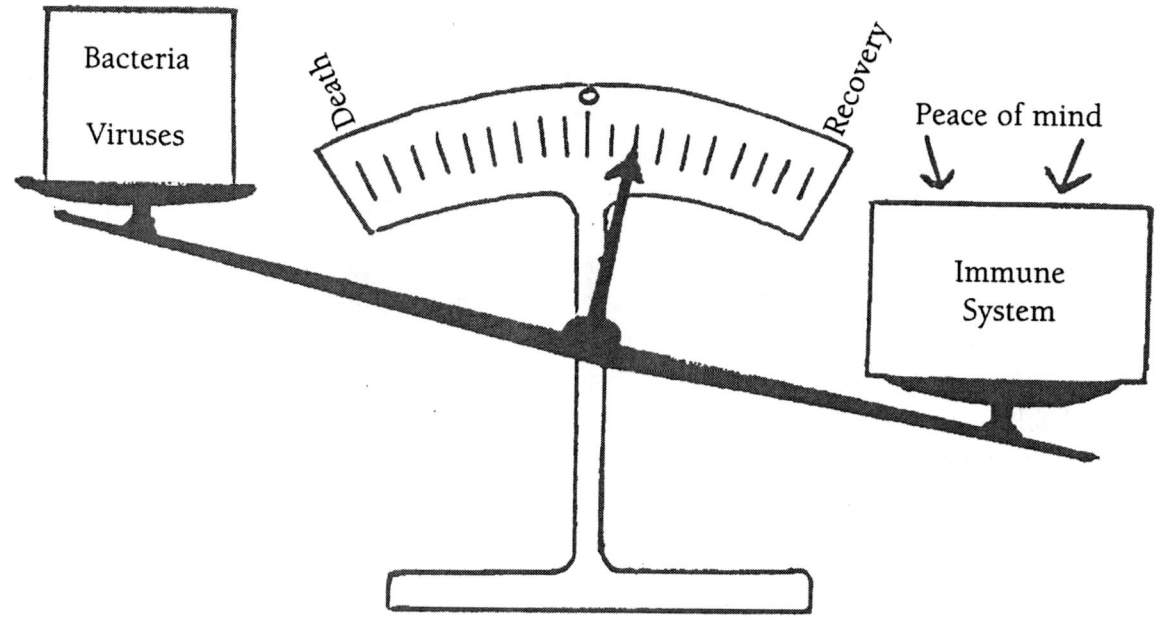

When resolution or healing of the painful or negative emotional problems takes place and peace is restored to the heart, this strengthens the immune system and can tip the balance toward recovery. This shows why emotional care, psychological support, and spiritual help can be of great benefit in helping persons recover from illness and be restored to wholeness.

This lesson teaches us another important principle. We now know that we are not just a victim of an illness, like tuberculosis, diabetes, or even AIDS. If we believe we are a victim of a disease, then we assume we can do nothing ourselves about it. Other than taking medicine and obeying the doctor's orders, we have no role to play in fighting the disease. However, we now know differently; there is indeed much we can do to fight against diseases. We can actually make our body and immune system stronger by doing the things discussed in this course. In this way, we are no longer 'victims' of a disease but are active participants in combating the illness and getting well.

Questions for reflection
1. List life-style issues and long-standing emotional problems that can affect health.

2. How do they contribute to illness?

3. How can we help them with these issues?

Now make it personal
1. When you have periods of contentment and tranquility in your life, how do you feel physically?

2. Think back on your own medical history. Remember times when you seemed especially susceptible to colds, the flu, or other illnesses. Do you see any connection between those times and times of particular stress?

3. Have you discovered ways to improve your ability to cope with stress?

Homework
1. Read *God, Medicine, and Miracles*, chapter 5
2. Read lesson 6 in *Helping Hurting People*

Lesson 6
The Architecture of the Heart
God, Medicine, and Miracles, *chapter 5*

We have talked much about the 'heart.' It is important now for us to understand what is in the heart, the inner self, so we will take a look at it. The heart is a big place with many things inside of it. Furthermore, much is taking place in our inner self all the time, day and night. In a very real sense, my heart is ME. It is WHO I am, and WHERE I am. I can function much better on a day-to-day basis if I have some understanding of WHO I am and of what is going on inside of me.

We can compare the heart, or the inner self, to a big house. Here is a drawing of a big house with many rooms. In each room are things that are in your heart, active things with constant interactions among them and a continuous influence over your body. Please understand that this is a very simplistic picture. We do not have walls, doors, windows, and rooms down inside of us. However, this illustration is a symbol of the inner self, and symbols can help us understand abstract concepts. In this case, the symbol can help us get a better grasp on the reality that is within us.

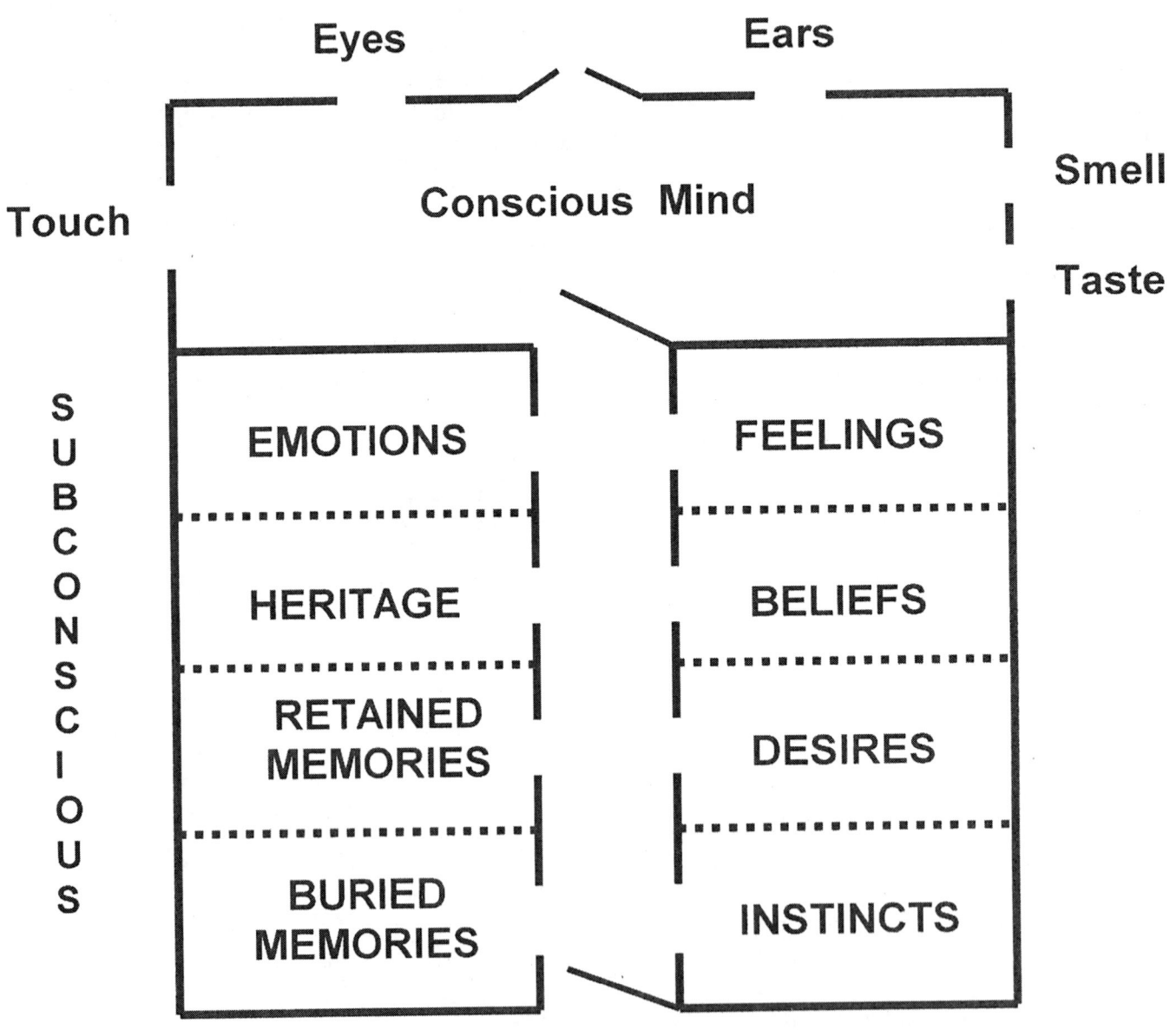

The Architecture of the Heart

The Conscious Mind
The conscious mind is where we have our thoughts, our reason, and our intellect. It is really a very small room because we can only think one thought at a time.

Many thoughts come into our conscious mind from the world around us. We have five 'windows' that allow things to come into the room of the conscious mind.
1. Eyes – our sight, that see things around us. You learn much through the 'window' of your eyes. This includes the many sights you see all the time, what you read, and what you see on television or the internet.
2. Ears – your hearing, as you listen to words and sounds. New thoughts come into your mind in class, as you hear other people talking, and as you listen to the phone, the radio or television.
3. Touch – You learn new thoughts as you feel things. You learn how things feel by touching them. You count the pulse or feel that a sick person is warm (has a fever).
4. Taste – You learn how different foods taste, and what spices make them taste better.
5. Smell – You learn the distinct odors that come from different things. The fragrance of a flower is pleasant; the odor of a skunk is terrible!

Just as thoughts come into your mind, so your thoughts go out of your mind to others. In our illustration here we say they go out the 'front door'. The front door is your speech, your gestures, and the different actions you perform to express yourself.

When you are awake, the conscious mind is a busy place. When you are asleep, it is quiet.

Subconscious mind
All that is below the room of the conscious mind is the subconscious mind. This is a big place, for many things are there. In the different rooms are your emotions, your feelings, your beliefs and desires, a multitude of memories of things past, the culture you have received from your parents, friends, and country, and the basic instincts that protect your life. We will look at what is in each of these rooms.

Between the conscious and the subconscious mind is a door that swings both ways. The thoughts in your conscious mind pass quickly into the subconscious mind to stimulate emotions, feelings and desires. They are stored there in the memory. Many things try to come from the subconscious mind 'up' into your thoughts and even go out through your words and actions. A strong emotion can burst out of the subconscious mind, go through the conscious mind quickly, and make you do or say things that may not be good before you have a chance to think about them. The conscious mind must control the door into the subconscious mind, slowing down bad feelings and emotions in order to handle them properly, and keeping bad thoughts from being stored in the memory.

Emotions
An emotion is an inner response to things that happen around us. You see or hear something, and this gives you a new thought. The thought goes down into the subconscious mind and is interpreted emotionally. If what you saw or heard makes you happy, you will have the emotion of joy. If what you saw or heard is a threat to you, you will have the emotions of fear or perhaps anger.

Emotions are a psychological energy that we can compare to a fire. Fire is an important part of life. It cooks our food, boils our water, and can make us warm. On the other hand, fire can burn or destroy us. The fire of joy makes us feel good and gives us the energy to do good things. The fire of anger is very strong. If you do not control it, anger can make you say harmful things or hurt other people. It is therefore important to control your emotions so that the heat and energy coming from them can help you do good rather than harm. Remember: each different emotion stimulates the brain to produce a specific neurochemical that influences all the organs of the body.

Feelings

Feelings are impressions you have about yourself and about things in the world around you. Some things make you feel good. Other things make you feel uncomfortable. Feelings are similar to emotions, but they last longer and are not as strong. They are more like a warm glow than an intense fire, a 'chill' rather than a sudden freeze. They also cause the brain to make neurochemicals that act on the organs of the body.

Beliefs

You have many beliefs in your heart, not just religious beliefs, but beliefs about everything. Beliefs are what you think is true, and what is of value. You believe certain things about yourself, your family, your country, your work, and the different things you do. Beliefs and values help you decide what you are going to do and how you are going to live. You do what you believe is good for you and of value to you. You have beliefs about morality, about actions that are good and helpful, and others that are bad and harmful.

Desires

Desires are in another 'room' in the heart. As persons, we desire to be happy, healthy, and strong. Often we desire to have power, to control other people, and to have power over the things around us. We have sexual desires: men have strong desires to be with women; women have strong desires to be with men. Most people have a strong desire for money and material possessions. These desires are like an inner energy. They push us to do certain things and to act in particular ways. You do many things in order to satisfy the desires of your heart.

Memories

You have two big rooms in your heart for memories. Think of these rooms as being full of filing cabinets. Each filing cabinet has many drawers, and each drawer contains many files. Everything that has happened to you from the time you were born is filed in a folder and is in a drawer in one of the filing cabinets.

Many events you can remember – recent events, and events that are important for you. These make up your available memories, for you can recall them to your thoughts. Many other events you have forgotten. You have forgotten almost all of the events that happened when you were a baby or a small child. You forget even more recent events if they are not important to you.

The Architecture of the Heart

The memories of some events are pleasant, but the memories of difficult ones may be painful. Even if you have forgotten a difficult event, the painful memory is still in your heart. It will not come into your thoughts, but will continue to influence your feelings, emotions, and desires. Memories cause the brain to make neurochemicals. A painful memory, even though buried in the subconscious mind, can cause your brain to make neurochemicals that can have a harmful effect on your body and make you ill.

Culture

Culture is an important part of the life of all of us. Culture is the collective attitudes, beliefs, and values of the people among whom we live. You have received many thoughts, beliefs, values, and feelings from your parents, your friends, your group, and your country. Much of what do is because you have learned to do this from your culture. These beliefs and values influence your thoughts, feelings, and desires. They influence the decisions you make about your life.

Instincts

In a room deep in your heart are what we call instincts. These are deep-seated, almost automatic responses to the basic needs of life. You have instincts to breathe air, eat food, drink water, and sleep when you are tired. You rarely think about these instincts, and you cannot really change them, for they are for your protection. You can suppress them for a short while, but you cannot change or eliminate them. Nor should you try.

Spirit

In this picture of the heart there is no single room for spirit. This is because your spirit is everywhere – in your thoughts, feelings, beliefs and values, memories, and so on. Spirit is the center of your whole self. It is your awareness of who you are, and it is where you are in contact with God or other spiritual powers.

The back door

At the end of the 'corridor' is a door. This door opens to the spiritual world in which you live. Through this door you can communicate with God. It is through this door the Lord comes into your heart when you invite him to come in. Or you communicate with other spiritual powers if you so wish. The handle of this door is only on the inside and is completely under your control. Not even God will force open this door if you keep it shut. Nor can evil spiritual powers. It is extremely important to guard this door carefully. Opening the door to harmful spiritual powers is dangerous. They can enter, install themselves in parts of your inner self, and take control over certain aspects of your personality.

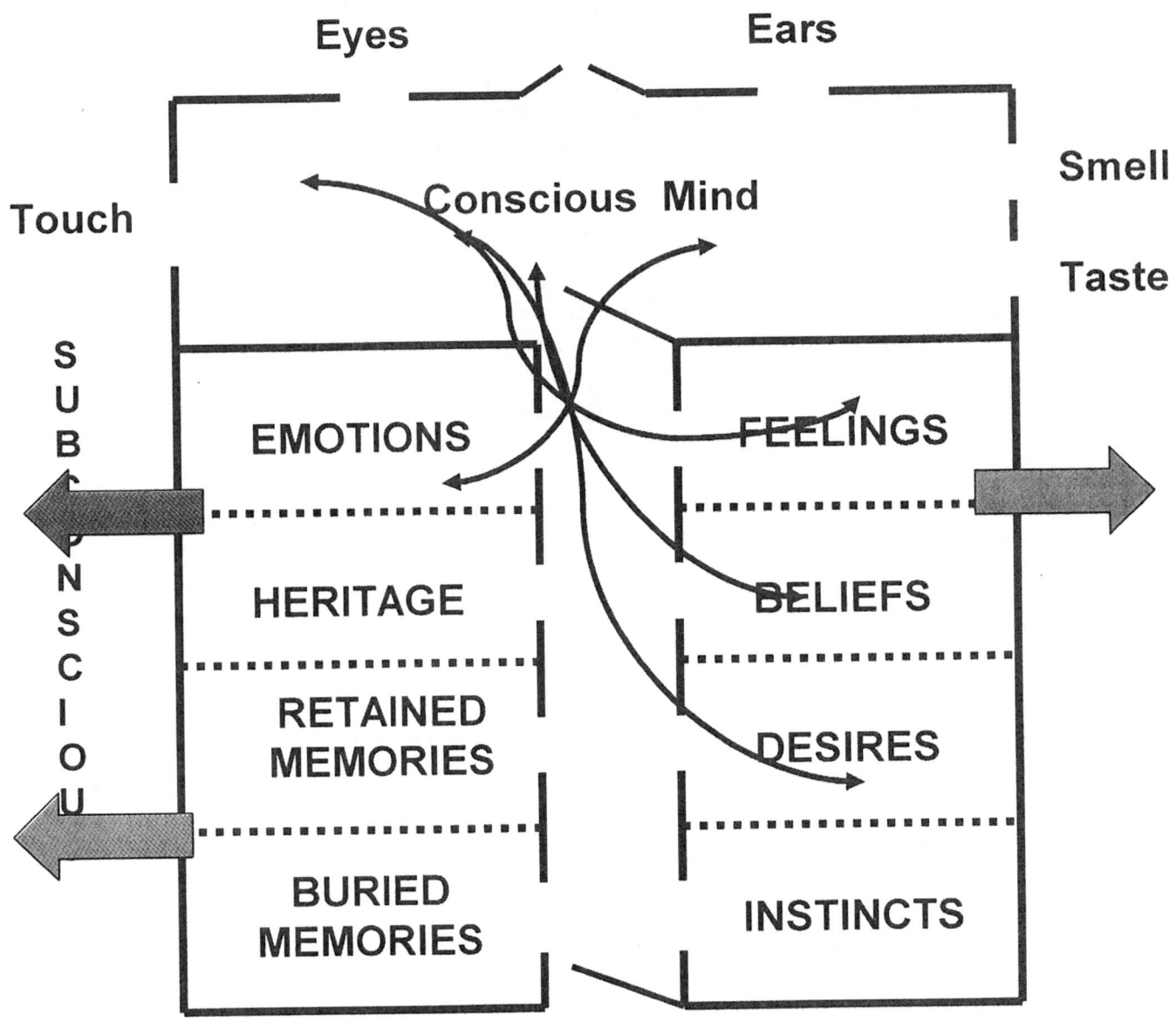

Summary

As you can see in the above diagram, all of the different things in the heart interact with each other. There are no real walls between them. Your emotions and feelings influence your thoughts, beliefs, desires, as well as your actions. Your memories affect your beliefs and values, your thoughts and feelings. We cannot separate the heart into special rooms as we have done in this picture. The whole heart functions as a unit, responding to what takes place in the world around.

The heart is also a part of the whole self. Through hormones and neurochemicals, it influences the whole body. Likewise, the sensations that occur in the body are communicated to the brain and stimulate thoughts, feelings, and emotions. Thus it is clear that we are whole persons with body, mind, and spirit functioning in a dynamic equilibrium.

Hygiene of the heart

It is very important to keep your heart in good order. If you allow yourself to see bad things or think bad thoughts, this will fill the rooms of your heart with harmful things. These negative thoughts and ideas will stimulate the brain to make neurochemicals that, over time, can make you ill. Certain types of negative thoughts, such as thoughts of violence or of sexual fantasies, have strong retentive power because they stimulate the production of powerful neurochemicals that are interpreted as pleasurable. This explains why these thoughts become compulsive and we become, in a sense, 'addicted' to them. On the other hand, if you see and hear good things, think good thoughts, and try to have good feelings and desires, you heart will be at peace. This in turn will make your body strong.

This is why the Apostle Paul said, "In conclusion, fill your minds with those things that are good and that deserve praise: things that are true, noble, right, pure, lovely, and honorable" Philippians 4 : 8. Such things are good not only for the soul but also for the health of the body.

Helping Hurting People

<u>Questions for reflection</u>
1. Think about a strong emotion you have had recently. Where did it come from? Did it affect you physically? If so, how? Try to describe this.

2. Can you remember a strong feeling you have had in the past? What effect did it have on you then? Could it be still affecting your subconscious mind, and perhaps even your body, now? If so, what can you do about it?

3. Why is it important to
   - screen incoming thoughts and impressions?

   - Control the swinging door between the conscious and subconscious minds?

<u>Homework</u>:
1. Read chapter 8 in *God, Medicine, and Miracles*
2. Read lesson 7 in *Helping Hurting People*

Lesson 7
Heart Problems That Affect Health
God, Medicine, and Miracles, Chapter 8

Now we will look at how problems in our conscious or subconscious mind can cause illness, even physical illnesses. We will see how some of the common feelings and emotions can produce symptoms of illness and look at examples of this. We will also see how Christ can bring resolution to many of these problems if we can bring to the hurting people his healing resources. Some examples are in the book *God, Medicine, and Miracles*, and to those you may be able to add examples from your experience.

Guilt
We are talking about the feeling of guilt. This is a deep feeling of remorse about something we have done. Sometimes the feeling of guilt is about something we have done *that is indeed wrong*. At other times it is about something we have done that *we believe is wrong* but may indeed not be wrong. In either case, the feeling is strong and can affect our physical health. It can cause inability to concentrate, loss of appetite, headaches, insomnia. What examples do you have from your own personal experience or from working with other people of the resolution of guilt?

Fear
Fear is a normal feeling that comes when we sense we are being threatened. It may be a real or an imaginary threat. Acute fear helps us protect ourselves. But retained fear can harm us. Such fear continues to stimulate the production of adrenalin and neurochemicals that keep our organs in a prolonged state of defense – heart, muscles, digestive system, etc. Eventually symptoms will develop: headaches, vague pains, palpitations of the heart, fatigue, vertigo, etc.

Anger
Anger is a normal emotion that comes when we feel evil attacking us or attacking those we care for. The moral aspect of anger is in how we handle it. We will look at this in more detail in lesson 17 as we study Ephesians 4: 26, 27. In that passage Paul tells us:
1. The will should control the intense emotion of anger. Otherwise, this psychological energy will lead us into saying or doing harmful things that we may later regret.
2. We should resolve quickly the problem that has stimulated the anger. If possible, we should resolve the conflict the same day.
3. Retained anger that smolders in the heart for months or years can cause many kinds of physical illnesses – hypertension, migraines, chronic inflammation in skin, joints, intestines, or elsewhere. In other words, chronic anger "gives the devil a chance" to make us sick.

Grudges and bitterness – the refusal to forgive another person
Grudges and bitterness do indeed 'poison' the spirit and can produce physical illness. They are associated with higher levels of circulating cortisol, the inflammatory hormone, and neurochemicals that, over time, can damage physical organs. They make people more susceptible to auto-immune diseases and can disturb cardio-vascular functions and digestion.

Think about how betrayal, divorce, abuse, or abandonment affect not only the feelings and emotions but can also influence one's health. How can we help a person whose heart is full of bitterness? We will look at that later as we discuss forgiving others.

Conflicting beliefs

Jesus said, "No one can serve two masters. Either he will hate the one and love the other, or he will be devoted to one and despise the other. You cannot serve both God and money" (Matthew 6: 24). Nevertheless, many people try to love two or more masters – God, money, prestige, pleasure, or other spiritual powers. The results are disastrous for mental health and even physical health.

Combining the Christian faith with the occult, or with greed (the Apostle Paul equates greed with idolatry), or with the worship of anything else can cause much inner conflict and anxiety. So also can the combination of high moral standards with unscrupulous behavior. These all can lead to physical problems of various sorts.

As Christians, it is essential that we avoid all contact or experience with the occult, including horoscopes, fortune tellers, mediums, the Ouija board, occult videos or games on TV or the internet, or any form of spiritism.

Painful experiences in the past: unresolved bad memories

Memories of trauma, tragedies, abuse, or conflicts can leave painful scars in the inner mind. The malaise and anxiety (often vague) from this can cause physical symptoms.

On pages 107 – 108 of *GMM* is the account of a young girl who suffered from severe pain with her monthly periods because of the painful memory of an abusive relationship. On pages 150 – 152 is a striking example of how a totally buried memory from prior to birth emotionally scarred a young man and caused a long-standing breathing disorder.

Reflect on this. Can you think of painful memories that have disturbed you and perhaps even caused physical symptoms? Jesus healed the terror buried in the heart of the young man who, at birth, felt he was suffocating. In the same way, Jesus can heal the painful emotions or feelings coming from any past events.

Compulsive behavior and addictions – *GMM*, chapter 9

An **addiction** is a condition of dependence upon an outside substance that the addict feels compelled to take in regularly in order to function. Such substances can be tobacco, alcohol, or drugs of various kinds.

In general, these substances replace normal neurochemicals produced by the brain. They suppress the production of these chemicals. Therefore, the body craves the outside substance because the brain no longer produces the normal neurochemicals. Sudden withdrawal of the addicting substance can cause severe and painful reactions for several days until the brain recovers the ability to produce the neurochemical again.

We have growing evidence that a dramatic spiritual experience can change neurochemistry and enable the brain to restart production of the suppressed neurochemical quickly.

Compulsive behavior patterns are similar to addictions. This is especially true in the area of sexual compulsions. Sexual pleasure stimulates the brain to produce neurochemicals called opioids. These opioids cause relaxation and diminish pain and stress for minutes or even hours. Opium is very similar to the normal opioids produced by the brain. This explains the powerful addicting effect of opium and heroin.

When a person engages in a pleasure-producing sexual activity, he experiences a surge of normal opioids that cause the body as well as the mind to feel good. When the opioid effect is finished, there is a normal desire to repeat the activity that gave such pleasure. The body craves the good feelings from the opioids. If the person repeats the activity on several occasions, he will become habituated to the surge of normal opioids. In other words, he becomes addicted to his own neurochemicals. This explains why compulsive sexual behaviors are extremely difficult to change. Here again, a dramatic spiritual experience can bring about such a change. [1]

On pages 155 – 159 of *God, Medicine, and Miracles* is the story of a Congolese physician who was set free from the power of three addictions and compulsive behavior. Consider how the addictions came about and how he was set free. Then look at other examples from your experience.

However, compulsive behavior and addictions are very complex entities. Many people struggle unsuccessfully to rid themselves of them. Working with them to help them find freedom is often a long and difficult task, and usually requires the help of professional counselors and/or support groups. We must avoid a simplistic approach to them while, at the same time, recognizing the power of God to intervene and bring healing and sharing with them the marvelous liberating resources Jesus has for us.

A Comprehensive Understanding of Illness

From this new understanding of illness, it becomes clear that illness and diseases can come from numerous areas of our life that may all be involved in making a person ill.

Physical disease
Illness can be primarily a *physical disease* such as trauma, infections, tumors, and so on. However, such diseases affect the emotions and stimulate fear, frustration, anxiety, etc. Diseases often disrupt social relationships and this further influences feelings and emotions. A serious disease can also affect the spirit, leading to depression, despair, and loss of hope. For example, the woman with bleeding in Mark 5 had a physical (gynecological) problem that affected her whole life and health.

Relational conflicts
Illness can come from *social conflicts*. A painful or broken relationship, divorce, violence, or abuse stimulate strong feelings of anger, grief, and fear. These can cause many physical problems – hypertension, headaches, stomach problems, certain allergies, auto-immune diseases, and many others.

Psychological problems
Illness can begin *in the mind or soul* - a real or imaginary guilt, shame, envy, fear or other negative feelings or emotions. If unresolved, these negative feelings and emotions can cause physical symptoms. The young man born with the umbilical cord around his neck and who suffered from a feeling of suffocation when he lay flat was ill because of the unresolved terror in his subconscious mind.

Spiritual problems

Illness can begin as a *spiritual problem*. Losing an important person or life support mechanism can lead to loss of hope, meaning, purpose, and the will to live. These can cause melancholy, depression, diminished appetite, and a weakened immune system that then opens the door for infections, cancer, and other physical problems.

From this it is clear that a team approach to healing is important.
1. Medical care to diagnose and deal with physical problems
2. Psychological care to discern problems of stress and negative emotions and to help a person find peace and joy.
3. Spiritual care to restore hope, meaning, and purpose

The story of John who nearly died of tuberculosis (*GMM* pages 35 – 38) is an excellent illustration of the comprehensive nature of illness. He had a physical disease in his lungs, but it did not respond to good medical treatment because of despair in his spirit and fear and anger in his feelings. These had so depressed his immune system that his body could not fight the infection even though he received the right antibiotics. Only when his soul and spirit were healed did his immune system regain its strength and he recovered from the infection.

In Mark chapter 2 we read the story of four men who brought their paralyzed friend to Jesus for healing. Mark says clearly that Jesus saw *their* faith and then healed the paralyzed man. We are like those four men. It is our faith that brings hurting people to Jesus. He is the one who does the healing. Let's not be negligent in bringing people to Jesus and accompanying them on their journey with him toward wellness.

[1] An excellent resource book for this is: *Homosexuality and the Politics of Truth*, by Jeffrey Satinover, Baker House, 1996

Heart Problems That Affect Health

Questions for reflection
1. How do these stories demonstrate that sickness involves the whole person?

2. What principles can we learn from them about how to bring healing to the inner person?

3. What resources can we offer to someone with a high level of fear?

4. What can we offer to a person who has much guilt (remorse) over a past act?

5. Someone has a painful memory of a traumatic event in childhood. How can we help them?

Homework:
1. Study Genesis chapter 2 : 16 – 17 : God's command to Adam, and all of chapter 3 – the story of the beginning of sin and its consequences.
2. Read *God, Medicine, and Miracles* – chapter 6
3. Read lesson 8 in *Helping Hurting People* and reflect on the questions at the end

Lesson 8
Sin and Its Consequences on Our Health
God, Medicine, and Miracles, Chapter 6

Sin is an uncomfortable word. Many people do not like it because it declares there is something wrong with us for which we are responsible. Where there is resistance to the word, we can talk about 'wrong-doing,' 'immoral behavior,' or "Have you done things you really regret?"

In any case, whatever we call it, sin or wrong-doing is related to illness. It offends that deep-seated sense of morality within us and stimulates the feeling of guilt. As we have seen, guilt can powerfully affect our health.

Sin and the presence of illness in the world

Read Genesis chapters 2 and 3. Here we find the story of the beginning of sin. Read also chapter 6 in *God, Medicine, and Miracles*.

What is sin?

Reflect on this story of sin and jot down what you think the Genesis account says about what sin is.

1.

2.

3.

What is the difference between 'sin' and 'sins'?

The consequences of sin are broken relationships. Now write down what the Genesis account says about the effect of sin on our relationships with:

<u>God.</u>   How does sin mess up our relationship with God, and why?

Self: How does sin mess up my relationship with my own inner self, and my self-esteem? What did that first act of disobedience do to the self-esteem of Adam and Eve?

Other people: Between man and woman. How did sin mess up gender relationships? The marriage bond?

How did it mess up all social relationships?

With the natural world
- How does sin diminish the fertility of the soil? See Genesis 3: 17 - 19
- The productivity of the land and the forests?
- The health of our water and the air we breathe?

How do all these disrupted relationships affect our health?

Illness can be a most profitable school master, teaching us valuable lessons about life in general and our personal life in particular. With some who have a chronic illness with which they are struggling, reflection on these questions can help them discover wisdom and even purpose in the illness

Read Psalm 103 : 1 – 5. Note the progression of ideas from verse one through verse five. Discuss the relationship of these ideas to each other, why they are arranged in that order, and what sin has to do with sickness and health. From this you can understand why we need to understand what sin is and how it can affect our health.

Personal sin and a particular illness

What is the relation, if any, between personal sin and illness? Medical science is uncomfortable with this question and rarely discusses it. Yet it is extremely important for us to understand the real relationship between sin and illness because our personal behavior is often implicated either in the origin of an illness or in our response to it, or both. We know that sickness has come into human life because of sin. Now we must think about the relationship between sin and the particular illness of a sick person. Basically there are four possibilities.

1. Certain personal sins can cause specific diseases
   - Sexually transmitted diseases
   - Substance abuse: tobacco, alcohol, drugs
   - Abuse of the body: overwork, overstress, over- or under-eating
   - Negligence of the body: poor nutrition, poor hygiene, lack of care

2. It may be the result of the sin of someone else.
   - Trauma, violence, war
   - Abuse by others
   - Neglect
   - Example: one third of HIV+ women in Africa have had only one sexual partner

3. There may be no relation whatsoever between the illness and personal sin.
   - Accidents happen
   - We live in a disease-filled world.

4. A sinful response to an illness may aggravate it, or impede the healing process.
   - Anger or resentment
   - Refusal to accept treatment, or help from others

Only the sick person can determine if sin is involved in his or her illness. God has not given us the right to accuse other persons of sin, no matter what they may have done. Only the Spirit of God can accuse someone of sin. However, because this is an important matter, we want to help sick persons deal with it and make changes that may be necessary to help them recover from the illness. Here are questions to ask that can enable a sick person to reflect on this issue.

Helpful questions we can ask sick persons

1. How is this illness affecting your life?
2. Do you sense that the illness is trying to teach you something:
   - About your life?
   - About things you may want to change: behavior, thoughts, reactions, emotions?
3. Are there things that have happened to you in the past that still trouble you?
4. Are there things you yourself have done that trouble you? Things you really regret?

The purpose of these questions is to help sick persons look at the illness in the context of their life, learn from it, and become stronger in dealing with it. We want to help them, in their minds, turn what they may feel is a tragedy into a challenge.

A sick person may describe to you things he has done, or is doing, that you consider to be wrong or sinful. You must never express your feelings about this, either by what you say or by facial expressions or gestures. On the other hand, you do want to help the person in this area, especially if it is affecting his health. What you can say is:
1. "Tell me how you feel about that," or
2. "How does (or did) this affect you, or your spouse, or others around you?"

In this way you are encouraging the person to think about past or present actions, and what these actions may be doing to his physical and emotional health, or doing to significant others in his life.

Principles to remember

1. We cannot accuse other persons of sin. They must come to this conclusion themselves.

2. Our role is simply to ask questions.

3. We do not want to give them a guilt trip. However, if their personal reflections do lead to a feeling of guilt, this can be healthy, for the cure for guilt is forgiveness.

4. All religions try to deal with sin. The approach of most religions is either to do penance for sin or to do many good works so that the overall balance between good and bad actions will be favorable. Christianity is the only faith that effectively deals with sin and its consequences by offering forgiveness and thus resolving the feeling of guilt. Jesus, by his death and resurrection, has not only dealt with the penalty of sin through forgiveness but gives us power to overcome it. We will now discuss this in detail.

5. The most powerful remedy for a deep sense of guilt is the word: "You are forgiven." We can pronounce forgiveness to anyone who confesses their sin to God. The authority for this is God himself, and the place we find it is in I John 1 : 9. Memorize this verse and have it available for anyone who truly needs to confess and be forgiven.

Sin and Its Consequences for Our Health

Questions for reflection
1. Write a brief paragraph on how sin does influence health.

2. Describe how, as caregivers, we can help people reflect on the issue of sin and their illness.

3. How can we gently offer them the true remedy for sin?

4. Think back on illnesses you have had. Do you see a connection between any of them and personal sin?

5. If so, how have you handled this? (Share this only if you feel comfortable in doing so.)

Homework
1. Read Exodus 15 : 22 – 26 and reflect on it. This is an event in the history of the Children of Israel, but also a powerful symbol for our own spiritual history.
2. Read lesson 9 in *Helping Hurting People*

Lesson 9
Salvation is Not Purification
God, Medicine, and Miracles, *chapter 7*

We sometimes assume that conversion, or coming into a personal relationship with Jesus, solves all our personal problems, resolves our inner burdens, and cures our spiritual malaise. It does not. Conversion and inner healing or purification are separate entities. However, conversion does bring into our spirit the One who can help us work through our problems, resolve inner conflicts, and heal any brokenness or wounds we may have in our spirit.

In Exodus 15 : 22 - 26 is a remarkable story that illustrates the difference between salvation and inner healing, and our need for both. We need to understand this story well, for it makes clear that salvation, or conversion, is only the beginning of a new life and that it makes available to us resources for healing and purifying our hearts. Here it is:

> Then Moses led the people of Israel away from the Red Sea into the desert of Shur. For three days they walked through the desert, but found no water. Then they came to a place called Marah, but the water there was so bitter that they could not drink it. That is why it was named Marah (Hebrew: 'bitter'). The people complained to Moses and asked, "What are we going to drink?" Moses prayed earnestly to the Lord, and the Lord showed him a piece of wood, which he threw into the water; and the water became fit to drink.
>
> There the Lord gave them laws to live by, and there he also tested them. He said, "If you will obey me completely by doing what I consider right and by keeping my commands, I will not punish you with any of the diseases that I brought on the Egyptians. I am the Lord, the one who heals you." [1]

As we examine this story we must remember:
1. The history of the Children of Israel is true a history. The events actually occurred.
2. Their history is also an allegory of our own spiritual history.
3. Therefore the historical events in the Old Testament have a meaning for us today.

Reflect on this story deeply and write down what the following mean for us today:
1. The slavery of the Children of Israel in Egypt.

2. The crossing of the Red Sea

3. The spring of water at Marah

4. The bitterness in the water

5. The piece of wood that God showed Moses

6. Why God tested the Children of Israel there

Notice the amazing progression here:

<u>Salvation</u> → <u>Inner healing</u> → <u>Obedience to God's commands</u> → <u>Health</u>

Yet how many of us fail to follow this progression? Our role as spiritual caregivers is to help hurting people see the full plan of life God has for us all, to determine where they are on this progression, and how they can continue to move forward in inner healing and obedience toward the health God wants them to have.

Conclusions

1. Salvation is an event to be followed by an on-going process of inner healing or purification in the deep mind or soul of the person.

2. Healing of the soul means freeing the person from the painful, negative, destructive emotions, feelings, and desires in the deep mind or soul of the person.

3. Healing of the soul is separate from salvation and is never complete in this life.

4. God has provided us with the means for both salvation and healing of the soul.

5. These should lead us into a life of obedience to the laws and commandments God has given us.

6. Obedience to God's laws favors health – physical, emotional, relational, and spiritual.

Salvation is Not Purification

<u>*Questions for reflection*</u>
1. What is the relationship between salvation and purification?

2. What is their relationship with obedience to God's will and commands?

3. How do these favor health?

4. How can you explain this story to people who have painful and negative emotions, feelings, and relationships?

<u>*Homework*</u>
1. Read Matthew chapters 26, 27, and 28 and reflect on what Jesus accomplished to deal with our sin and to make available to us important resources for our healing.
2. Then read *God, Medicine, and Miracles* chapter 7.
3. Read lesson 10 in *Helping Hurting People*

[1] "I am the Lord, the one who heals you." – Jehovah Rapha

Lesson 10
What Did Jesus Accomplish for Our Healing?
God, Medicine, and Miracles, – Chapter 7

    The word Jesus comes from the Hebrew word YESHUWAH which means both savior and healer. Modern Christianity emphasizes Jesus as our Savior, and our need for salvation. He is indeed our Savior from the penalty and the power of sin. However, we ignore or have forgotten that he is also a Healer, that he came to heal the broken heart and the wounded spirit, and that we all need his healing power.

    Three events in Jesus' ministry are crucial for our healing. By these events, he has made available to us potent resources for the healing of the heart and the spirit. Think deeply about these events before looking at the accompanying video. The first event took place in the Garden of Gethsemane.

The Garden of Gethsemane – Matt. 26: 36 – 46; cf Luke 22: 39 – 44

    Then Jesus went with his disciples to a place called Gethsemane, and he said to them, "Sit here while I go over there and pray." He took with him Peter and the two sons of Zebedee. Grief and anguish overcame him, and he said to them, "The sorrow in my heart is so great that it almost crushes me. Stay here and keep watch with me."

    He went a little further on, threw himself face downward on the ground, and prayed, "My Father, if it is possible, take this cup of suffering from me! Yet not what I want, but what you want."

    Then he returned to the three disciples and found them asleep, and he said to Peter, "How is it that you three were not able to keep watch with me for even one hour? Keep watch and pray that you will not fall into temptation. The spirit is willing, but the flesh is weak."

Once more Jesus went away and prayed, "My Father, if this cup of suffering cannot be taken away unless I drink it, your will be done." He returned once more and found the disciples asleep; they could not keep their eyes open.

    Again Jesus left them, and prayed the third time, saying the same words. Then he returned to his disciples and said, "Are you still sleeping and resting? Look! The hour has come for the son of Man to be handed over to the power of sinful men. Get up; let us go. Look, here is the man who is betraying me!"

1. Why was Jesus in such anguish of soul?

2. What was he facing that was so repulsive to him?

3. What did he actually do in the Garden?

4. Why is this so important for our healing?

The Cross
1. Jesus was nailed to the cross at 9 AM. He died 6 hours later at 3 PM.

2. Normally it takes from 24 to 72 hours for a crucified man to die on the cross. Death comes from exhaustion and asphyxia. Jesus did not die of asphyxia because, at the final moment, he cried out with a loud voice. Someone suffocating cannot do that.

3. Why did Jesus die so quickly? – in just 6 hours?

4. What was the physical cause of his death?

5. What was the real cause of his death?

6. How can an understanding of this help heal the heart and spirit?

The empty tomb – Mark 16: 1 – 9
1. What message does Jesus' resurrection speak to our hearts?

2. Why is it important to know that the tomb was empty?

3. The empty tomb is the symbol that gives us true hope. Peter calls it our "living hope" (I Peter 1 : 3). What does "living hope" mean for us?

In these accounts we find great power for healing the broken heart and the wounded spirit.
1. In many cultures and throughout the Bible, blood is a powerful symbol. It is a symbol of life, and the shedding of blood signifies death. God told the people of Israel that forgiveness of sin requires a blood sacrifice. This means something had to die because of a person's sin. God did this to impress on peoples' hearts the seriousness of sin.
2. However, the sacrifice of an animal for sin was too cheap, and the symbolic effect too weak. God, therefore, has provided a far more powerful symbol for forgiveness, his own blood, because Jesus is God in human flesh. God now says to our broken and guilty hearts: "I died for you. It is *my* blood that was shed for your sin. It is sufficient."
3. Sin, therefore, is extremely serious. It cost God the blood of his Son.

4. The guilt in our hearts because of sin can be very heavy. Yet the message is clear: the power of the blood of Jesus Christ is greater than the horribleness of any sin that we can possibly commit, and of the sins of everyone in the world, because Jesus came back to life. Sin could not overcome Jesus because the power of his life is greater.
5. When we accept what Jesus has done for us and ask him to enter our hearts and make his overcoming power available to us, this not only saves us but can heal the wounds sin has made in our hearts and give us the power to deal with sin in the future.

<u>The healing power of these stories</u>

When it is appropriate, you can tell a sick person what Jesus did for him in the Garden of Gethsemane. He actually took into his own spirit all the evil powers that have such a strong influence on our lives, and all of the sins we commit. You may want to mention the particular sins of this person or the evil powers he is dealing with. Tell him that Jesus <u>voluntarily</u> accepted these things in order to carry them to the cross. The cross itself did not kill Jesus. Rather it was the incredible weight of the sin and evil in his heart that broke his heart and killed him. They killed him because he, willingly and for our sake, allowed them to kill him so that they would not have to kill you or any of us who believe in him.

Powerful as these evil things are, and however frightful was his death, Jesus did not stay dead. He rose again to life on Sunday morning because the power of his life is greater that the combined power of sin, evil, and death. His healing and life-giving power is now available to you. The stories we have already told illustrate how what Jesus did in Gethsemane and on the cross can heal the wounded spirit of a hurting person. Explaining these stories of Jesus to a person struggling with conflicts, guilt, or other forms of anguish can be of immense benefit for healing. In the next section we will discuss how to apply his healing resources in a clinical setting to people with specific inner problems.

Helping Hurting People

Questions for reflection

1. Why is it so important to explain to hurting people the healing power of Jesus and invite them to accept it?

2. How does Jesus truly heal the broken heart and wounded spirit?

3. What effect can this have on physical illnesses?

Homework

1. Now look at the DVD lesson: *Jesus in Gethsemane*
2. Then read lesson 11 in *Helping Hurting People*
3. And read the appendix in *God, Medicine, and Miracles*

Lesson 11
Establishing a Caring Relationship

A caring relationship is one that is open, sincere, and shows genuine interest in the other person. All health professionals, from a highly trained specialist to a patient advocate to a receptionist, should be able to demonstrate compassionate care expressed in a caring relationship. What does a caring relationship look like?

Take a moment to think back on a time when you were sick, or grieving, or hurting inside for some other reason. Did someone come alongside of you whom you found to be helpful? If so, what was it about her, him, or them that was especially helpful to you? Write down a list of the attitudes, words said, and caring acts done by that person or those helpers. If you are in a group, discuss these things among you.

Now consider the opposite. Were there others who came to you who were not helpful, or who maybe even made you feel worse? If so, jot down the unhelpful things they said or did and discuss them. Now let's look at a list of the attitudes that demonstrate a caring spirit.

Attitudes a caregiver must have

<u>Compassion</u> means 'to feel with.' We attempt to feel what another person is feeling. When a person is suffering, we try to show more by our gestures than by our words that we want to understand, or enter into, what he or she is feeling.

<u>Accepting</u>. A few sick persons are difficult to accept as persons. They may be weak, poor, have a bad odor, or come from a different social group. We must accept each one as a real person and affirm him or her as a person of great value. Jesus did that. He even touched persons with leprosy. This is essential for caring, and we must do the same.

<u>Gentleness</u>. This means speaking softly, kindly, and without criticism or judgment. Often we hear sick persons describe bad things in their life. We can ask them how they feel about this, but should not tell them that it is bad. They must come to recognize that themselves.

<u>Sincerity</u>. We must show genuine interest in what a person is telling us and express a willingness to be helpful to them. We cannot simply pretend to be interested or to want to help, for if we just pretend to be interested, the sick person will realize this quickly and will have no confidence in us.

<u>Keeping a secret</u>. When sick persons tell us their problems, we have no right to tell those problems to someone else. In class when you are talking about a sick person you know, do not use his name or give other information that will enable others to know who you are describing.

Never be brutal, abrupt, or rude to a sick person. Words can harm the soul and spirit of other persons. So be careful what you say to them. Always speak kindly.

Helping Hurting People

Principles to Follow

In order to establish and maintain a caring relationship with hurting people, there are certain principles to follow.

Observation

The first important principle to master is to *observe* the hurting person – posture, facial expressions, and tone of voice. Look for signs of
1. depression or grieving: sitting slumped forward, speaking slowly, indistinctly, in monosyllables, or not speaking at all.
2. nervousness – fidgeting, fingering objects, rapid shaking of a foot or leg, constantly looking at one's watch, tics
3. worry or fear – distracted gaze, fearful facial expression, frequent changes of position

A brief comment on your part can be helpful, such as "You look sad, or worried, or anxious." A statement of this nature is less threatening than a question asking, "Are you sad, of worried, or anxious?" That could put a person on the defensive.

On the other hand, it may be more appropriate to say nothing at this point about what you observe. However, make a mental note of it, for this can guide you as you proceed further in discerning the real problems of the hurting person.

Non-verbal communication

A second important principle to remember is that much of what we communicate to another person is done non-verbally, by gestures, facial expressions, posture, and so forth. We need to understand this and then to learn how to put into practice non-verbal expressions of interest, sympathy, and a desire to help. Here is an important list of the non-verbal ways we send messages to other people.

Posture

An open posture conveys interest; a closed posture expresses indifference or even animosity. How do you maintain an open posture?
1. Lean slightly toward the other person.
2. Keep both arms and hands in your lap or on the arms of your chair. Crossing your arms sends a clear signal: "I'm not interested in what you are saying."
3. Keep both feet on the floor. Crossing your legs is another signal of disinterest.
4. Relax. Constant fidgeting, fingering a set of keys or another object, drumming on the chair arm, or shaking a foot or leg, are distracting movements and indicate nervousness or preoccupation elsewhere. You want the hurting person to relax and feel at ease. This is possible only if you are at ease.
5. Face toward the other person, with no desk, table, or other furniture in between.

Distance

All of us instinctively want a certain space around us. If another person comes too close, we feel uncomfortable. On the other hand, if a person sits too far from us, this conveys a lack of interest or even a judgmental spirit. The appropriate distance to sit from a hurting person requires a bit of intuition. It is important to be close enough to convey interest and concern but not so close as to make the person feel uncomfortable or threatened. It is better to begin the conversation sitting at a distance that is comfortable for you, with the option of moving closer if that seems appropriate.

Facial expressions

Relax your facial muscles. A smile conveys warmth, contentment, and approval, although it can be inappropriate if the person is grieving, angry, or in pain. Avoid facial tension, involuntary movements, furrowed brows, or any other indication of impatience, criticism, or anger. Stifle any desire to yawn, but if a sneeze or yawn slips out, excuse yourself appropriately and move on. A nod of the head, a raised eyebrow, and a slight smile can encourage a person to continue talking. This also assures the person you are listening.

Eye contact

In most cases, looking at the other person conveys a message of interest and concern. Some people, however, are uncomfortable with eye contact, so you must respect that. When the hurting person does make eye contact with you, acknowledge it by a brief smile, or nod as an encouragement to proceed.

Voice

This includes both tone and volume. You must adjust the volume of your voice so the other person can hear you clearly, but not raise it above the necessary level. The tone of your voice should be gentle, not harsh, and never brutal. Adjust the speed of talking so the person can follow you easily, but avoid speaking too slowly. This would diminish the interest of the other person in what you are saying.

Gestures

Avoid unnecessary gestures of hands and arms. If you have a tendency to talk like a windmill, make an effort to ratchet down the maneuvers of your arms, for this can create distraction and discomfort. Never pick your nose, bite or file your fingernails, or screwdriver your ear. On the other hand, extending a hand, indicating approval or a question by a gesture, these can be helpful.

Touching

You may be a "touchy-feely" person, often reaching out to other persons to grasp a hand or place your hand on their arm. That may be appropriate for you, but often it is not for a hurting person. A non-touchy-feely person may feel uncomfortable or even threatened by such a gesture. It is far better to err on the side of being too conservative (not touching) than being too forward.

<u>Asking questions</u>

A good question is like a key opening a door. It enables the person to express herself. A good question is an *open* question that cannot be answered simply by a yes or no. Rather, it allows the person to talk about the subject and say whatever she wishes to say. For example:
1. What brings you to see the doctor?
2. How long have you been ill?
3. Or even, tell me about your illness.

Encouraging the person to describe the illness is often a good way to begin the conversation, for it shows your interest and is a non-threatening subject. Do not ask for details because that is the domain of the health care provider. However, use what the person describes about the illness as a point of departure into more personal matters.

To begin talking about more personal issues you can ask or say:
1. How are things going at home, or at work, or in school?
2. Are you carrying a heavy load of stress?
3. What stressful situations are of concern to you, or
4. Are there personal relationships that are difficult for you at this time?

Avoid threatening or judgmental questions, especially the question Why?
1. Why did you do that?
2. Why do you feel this way?
3. Why did you let yourself get into this situation?

Such questions put a person on the defensive and make free expression more difficult.

Do not ask negative questions, such as "Didn't you feel like you had done wrong?" Negative questions are ambiguous, both in the question and in the answer. A No answer could mean either, "No, I didn't" or "No. I did feel that way." In either case, further clarification is needed. So phrase questions positively.

<u>Listening</u>

Listening attentively is an essential skill for this ministry. It is a skill that can be learned by practice and by a disciplined focus on what the other person is saying. In the story told in Mark 5 of Jesus and the woman with chronic bleeding, Mark says, 'She came trembling with fear, fell at his feet, and told him the whole story.' Although Mark does not say it, we can be sure that Jesus listened attentively.

Listening, by itself, is therapeutic. If you have created a 'safe environment' of trust and listen carefully, the relief of unburdening or of sharing a deep concern can have a genuine healing effect. If you have a tendency to 'butt in' when another person is speaking, train your self out of it. Monitor your casual conversations at home, at work, or with friends, and make a conscious effort to avoid interrupting. Ask your spouse or a close friend to help you, for so often we do it unconsciously. Allowing a person to finish what she is saying and complete a story or a train of thought, is polite and affirming. Interruptions are actually attempts on our part to 'break in and steal,' selfish efforts to steal the spotlight and control the conversation.

So listen without interruption. Allow the person to continue talking until she seems to be finished. Nothing is more disconcerting to a person trying to tell a story or to express a concern than for someone to interrupt and try to change the train of thought. However, occasionally interjecting, "Yes, I see," or "That makes sense," or "Tell me more" can encourage the person to continue sharing her story.

Establishing a Caring Relationship

Listen to the content of what the person is saying. If it is not clear, an occasional interruption for clarification may be indicated, such as: "I did not quite understand you there." Or "I am not sure of what you are telling me; please go over it again." If your thoughts do wander and you miss something you think may be important, simply say, "Could you please repeat that? I did not hear it very well."

A tendency many of us have while another person is speaking is to begin formulating what we want to say when our turn comes. This seriously damages the caring relationship, for our thoughts are not on what the person is saying. Usually the person is aware of that and so thinks 'You are not really listening to me.'

As the person is talking, make a mental note of ideas or events you feel are important to pursue. You can even jot down a word or two to help you recall a particular concern. In general, however, avoid taking extensive notes, for this can turn a caring relationship into an interview.

<u>Observe the person carefully</u> while she is talking: facial expressions, posture, tone of voice, a catch in the voice, tears forming, or signs of nervousness. These can be indications of an underlying problem. Short periods of silence can be significant, so when the person pauses, don't jump in quickly with a question or comment. A brief, "Yes, I understand," or "Is there more you want to say about this?" can help a person continue if she so desires.

<u>Discerning and reflecting feelings</u>

This is a simple statement you make in order to clarify what the person is feeling. As she is describing a situation, or telling the story of an event, try to discern what she is really feeling. You can then say: "That must have made you feel really good! or sad; or angry," or "I can imagine that you felt scared to death!"

Your perception of her feelings may be incorrect, but that does not matter. Your statement will affirm your concern for her. She may not have felt the way you thought she did. So she will correct your impression and clarify for you how she really felt if indeed she herself knows. If she is uncertain of her feelings, this will help her reflect on what has been going on in her feelings and emotions.

Occasions will occur when you do not know what to say next. A statement to try to reflect feelings may be useful at this point: "I sense you have really been feeling lonely... or rejected... or anxious..." or "It sounds to me like you were feeling guilty about that."

You can also help a person clarify her story or her feelings by saying, "What I am hearing you say is.......... Is that really so?" It may not be so, but this will allow the person to restate or perhaps rethink what she has been saying.

<u>Responding to emotions</u>

You will encounter a broad spectrum of emotions as you work with hurting people. It is of utmost importance that you keep your emotions under control and be able to respond appropriately both verbally and emotionally.

Weeping is the normal expression of the emotion of grief. The tear glands are our organs of elimination of grief, and weeping can be healing. When a hurting person weeps in your presence, do not be embarrassed, and never respond by saying, "Don't cry." Sit quietly, with an open posture, and wait. Use the time to pray silently. If appropriate and you feel led, placing your hand on her arm or shoulder can convey support and comfort.

On the other hand, if a hurting person expresses anger at the health system or even at you, do not respond with anger or by defending yourself or the system. Remember that the person is suffering and may be angry at the illness, frustrated by the circumstances, or even angry with God. There may also be genuine cause for anger against the health system. Nevertheless, a gentle response such as, "Yes, I know you have been suffering, or that bad things have happened. I hope we can talk about this so I can try to be helpful to you."

Never express judgment, criticism, or condemnation, no matter what you hear. If a man says he has abused his child, wait gently for him to continue his story. If he does not, ask simply, "Would you like to tell me more about this?" Or, "How do you feel about it?" Show no sign of disapproval, no matter how terrible the event appears to be. Any suggestion of condemnation on your part will make it more difficult for you to be of any help to him.

<u>Empowering</u>
None of us, either health providers or spiritual caregivers, can solve the problems of hurting people. Nor should we even suggest possible solutions, for they would be our solutions and not theirs. However, by careful questions about options and the positive and negative aspects of each one, we can encourage people in their search for wisdom and help. The only one who can give true guidance and the needed on-going support is the Lord himself.

Our role is to stimulate reflection and prayer, to encourage and support, and to empower hurting people to respond creatively to the challenges they face with the help of the Lord. In no way, however, do we want to build an unhealthy dependency of hurting persons on us as caregivers. This is not good for them, nor for us.

On the other hand, during periods of special need – the death of a spouse, a recent divorce, a significant loss – a person may need a supportive friend who can give on-going comfort, encouragement, and even guidance. Good judgment is necessary, however, to discern to what extent and for how long this should continue. But it may be lifesaving to a hurting person until such time as emotional and spiritual strength returns and new relationships are built.

<u>Referral to a professional counseling service</u>
Certain conditions merit professional counseling
1. The possibility of the sick person harming himself or another person
2. Signs of serious depression
3. Complex emotional or spiritual issues that require professional assistance

Establishing a Caring Relationship

In general it is the physician, not the spiritual caregiver, who makes the referral. When you, as the spiritual caregiver, believe that the person you are trying to help could benefit from the help of a professional counselor, it is often wise to suggest this to the person and describe the benefits of such counseling. If the person seems open to this and has the means to do so, suggest that the person discuss referral with the physician or, if he or she prefers, to give you permission to suggest it.

If the sick person does not want professional counseling, or cannot afford it, yet the person could harm himself or someone else, then you must inform the physician of these concerns. The physician can then assume the responsibility for doing what is necessary to protect the person and others from harm.

Confidentiality

The basic rule of confidentiality is that every conversation with a sick person, every observation, and all impressions must be kept secret. The story of a sick person belongs to her. She has shared it with you because she wants your help. However, she has not given you ownership over it. If you now pass her story on to someone else, you have, in fact, stolen her story, and that is unethical. Furthermore, word will quickly circulate that you are not a person in whom one can confide. It is wise, at the beginning of the relationship, to assure the person that everything she says will be kept confidential.

There are, however, exceptions to this rule.
1. The person herself may give you permission to share part or all of her story with someone else, such as the health provider.
2. The person has told you something that poses a danger to herself, such as the desire to commit suicide. This needs to be reported immediately to your superior, or to the health provider, because such a person needs help right away.
3. The person has indicated she wants to harm or has harmed someone else. This also must be reported in order to protect the other person.

If you are not sure if you should report a conversation or impression, discuss this with your supervisor or health provider, but do it anonymously at first as you ask for advice. We must not betray confidences. On the other hand, we must not be an accomplice to those who would harm themselves or others.

Getting started

A certain degree of nervousness as you begin this ministry is very normal. You are in a new situation. You will be meeting new people. You will be using new skills and needing new wisdom. You may think this is scary. In reality, however, it is healthy to be fearful for it encourages you to seek God's help and trust in the sufficiency of his grace. It will come, for this is God's work to which he has called you, and he will be present with you.

It also means that you should make prayer your habit: praying each day before you begin, as you are with hurting people, and as you finish. Pray also for the other members of the team, and pray for those who will be coming to talk with you. If possible, ask a few close friends to pray regularly with you and for you, as a prayer support group. Then when you have prayed and know that others are praying for you, simply trust. When Jesus was on his way to the house of Jairus to see Jairus' sick daughter, word came that the daughter had died. Jesus said quietly to Jairus, "Don't be afraid. Just trust me." Those are marvelous words as we do the work of Jesus. We can simply trust him.

<u>Suggestions</u>:
1. As you are conversing casually with others – spouse, friends, colleagues, or sick people – try to pay attention to how you sit or stand, your posture, tone of voice, distance, and gestures. Pay attention also to eye contact – do you make it appropriately? And your facial expressions – what do they convey?

2. Monitor how you listen to your spouse or friends. Do you listen without interrupting, or do you have a tendency to break into the middle of what someone else is saying?

3. Observe the non-verbal messages you receive from others in casual conversations. What messages do you notice from your spouse or from a close friend?

4. Do you have any nervous or distracting gestures that may interfere with good communication? – nail biting, fidgeting, handling an object like keys, etc.

So pay attention to the communications in which you are involved and that are occurring around you. Try to improve your own communication methods and attitudes to make them as effective and helpful as possible.

Establishing a Caring Relationship

Questions for reflection
1. What non-verbal messages that others send you really bother you?

2. How can you perceive attitudes others may have toward you?

3. How can you tell whether or not another person is listening to you? Or is interested in you?

4. What kind of questions can encourage people to talk?

5. What are appropriate ways to handle emotions others express, like
   - Anger?

   - Weeping?

Homework
Read lesson 12 in *Helping Hurting People* on How to Do a Personal Assessment

Lesson 12
Personal Assessment

To understand better what is happening in the lives of sick persons, we must listen to their story. This is important for health professionals; it is likewise important for the spiritual caregivers. This general outline needs to be in your mind as you listen to sick persons. A few short questions can often uncover personal problems that may need attention. You will never ask all of these questions of any one person. However, it is good to have them available in your mind to ask when a particular question is appropriate. Start in a way that puts the hurting person at ease. For example: "You have told me about your illness. So tell me about yourself." Start with general questions like these:

General
1. How are things going in your life?
2. Any problems at work? At home? At school?
3. How are you coping with this illness?
4. To whom can you go for help in time of need?

Relationships
Relationships are a major part of our lives, and strongly influence our inner life, our thoughts, feelings, and emotions. These questions about relationships can give you an idea of what is happening in the life of the person.
1. Are you having problems with your spouse, your children, your parents?
2. Are you having problems with someone at work, or at school?
3. Is there anyone else you are having difficulty getting along with? Or who has offended you? Or who is making your life miserable?
4. Do you have trouble making friends? Does this concern you?
5. Do you have a problem with someone of the opposite gender?
6. Are you having trouble with your own self-confidence?

Level of Stress
Find out how much stress the person is facing, and, more importantly, how he or she is handling it.
1. Do you feel you are under much pressure? If so, from what?
2. Do you feel down in your spirit, or depressed?
3. Do you feel nervous or tense about anything?
4. Are you having difficulty in concentrating, or getting work done?
5. Are you having trouble sleeping?
6. How are you eating? Are you losing the desire to eat? Or eating too much?
7. Any problems with employment? Or finances? Or another aspect of living?

Recent loss
Loss of important people or major support structures can be devastating. Ask about this.
1. Have you recently lost a close relative or friend?

2. Are you going through a separation or divorce?
3. Have you lost your job, or are you afraid you might do so?
4. Have you retired? If so, how is that going? What now interests you?

Habits

Compulsive habits or addictions have serious consequences for health. Find out about this and also, where a problem exists, if the person wants help with it. Many of these habits are complex, and expert help is often needed in dealing with them.
1. Are you having a problem with smoking? Or drinking? Or using drugs? If so, would you like help with this?
2. Is gambling a concern for you?
3. Are there any other habits you are struggling with and would like help with?

For a young person

The present nature of our culture can have devastating effects on young people. Broken families, the constant impact of the media, strong peer pressures, and confusing messages present many difficulties to children and young people. Ask gentle but penetrating questions to try to discern if a young person is struggling with major issues.
1. Where are you heading in life?
2. What would you really like to be?
3. Do you feel like you are getting what you desire out of life?
4. Have you ever really thought about who you are?
5. Are you facing pressure from peers or others that is difficult for you?

These questions are designed to open up any areas of concern a person may have. The questions are not threatening but give sick persons the opportunity to talk about a particular concern if they wish to. The questions also demonstrate your interest in the person and in determining the various areas of need.

It is by no means necessary to ask all of these questions with everyone. But when the answer to one question in a category is positive, it may be wise to ask the other questions in that area. If a serious issue comes up, you may feel it wise to pursue that concern and leave the remainder of the questions or other areas of life for a later time.

In addition to these questions, the computerized intake exam form may give you significant information. Look for items about religious affiliation or preference, contact persons, habits that may be deleterious to health, etc. A question about any of these items may open the door to problem areas or to spiritual issues.

A sick person may object to this, considering it as prying into his or her personal life. Or one may say, "Are you implying that my illness is all in my head?" Here a brief explanation of wholeness can be helpful. Medical science is now aware that our personal feelings do affect the heart, blood pressure, the digestive system and, in reality, the whole body. An understanding of personal concerns and stress levels can facilitate a more comprehensive approach to care and a more rapid recovery.

Personal Assessment

Many people have difficulty talking about their past history. They are reserved and do not share their lives with others. The personal and spiritual questions we ask may make them uncomfortable. In such cases, it may be possible for the spiritual caregiver to help a person tell his or her story by adopting a more conversational mode and asking open non-threatening questions. Here is an example of what a spiritual caregiver can do:

1. Where did you grow up? After listening, you can say, "I grew up in such-and-such a place."
2. What was your town like?
3. Did you go to a good school? Then, "Yes, I remember being in such-and-such a grade and how it went."
4. What did you Dad do? Did your Mom work?
5. Were there tough times back then?

This can then lead into questions about difficult experiences that are still painful and may be influencing the person's life and health now.

Experiences early in our lives can have a profound influence on us and on our health. Traumatic events in childhood or adolescence affect us deeply. These can be emotional trauma, physical or emotional abuse, the death of a parent or sibling, divorce, and other serious upheaval in life. The story of an important failure, an abortion, or a misdemeanor may come out. We can then begin to see where real problem areas lie and ask God's help silently for wisdom in helping the person bring these problem areas to the Lord for healing. We will discuss this in more detail as we proceed.

Questions for reflection

1. What is a good way to keep these questions in mind, or at hand, so that you can ask the ones that are appropriate with a hurting person?

2. Some people are reticent and do not open up easily to talk about themselves. What are possible ways to help people begin to talk about themselves?

Homework
Read lesson 13 in *Helping Hurting People* on Taking a Spiritual History

Lesson 13
Taking a Spiritual History

Up until recently it was considered unethical to talk about spirituality and particularly about Jesus in the clinic. This has now changed. Over the past two decades a large volume of medical literature about spirituality has developed with more than 800 articles published describing the interface between religion and health. The great majority of these studies demonstrate scientifically that religion and spiritual activities have a beneficial effect on health and on recovery from illness. Since these studies make clear that spirituality is a factor in health and recovery, it is now ethical to ask questions of sick persons about their spiritual life. We can even consider it unethical not to ask questions about spiritual issues.

It must be done with great care, however. This is a delicate matter which requires tact, gentleness, and flexibility. You may care for persons who have other faiths or claim no religion at all. We must respect every person of whatever faith they have and encourage their spiritual growth in every way possible.

Here are principles to remember:
1. Faith in general has positive effects for health and for healing. As we have seen, faith in Christ has special benefits for both.
2. Imposition of one's personal faith, manipulation of the beliefs of the sick person, and any pressure to change beliefs, religious or church affiliation, or ways of worship must be avoided in all circumstances. This is called "proselytism" and is unethical.
3. We can, however, offer to discuss faith in Christ with the person *if he or she wishes*.
4. If the sick person is not interested in the Christian faith or resists it, we go no further with the discussion. However, we should make every effort to maintain a caring relationship with the person so as to continue to be of any possible help to him or her.

The timing of asking about faith is variable and requires discernment. In general, it should come only after:
1. a relationship of openness and confidence has been established
2. the sick person has described the illness
3. we have asked questions about family, work, and personal life
4. social, emotional, or spiritual problems related to the illness or to personal life have surfaced.

A good rule to follow is this: Don't hurry, but be alert to hints or comments that can be door openers to the area of spiritual life. When you feel the time is appropriate to do a spiritual assessment, here are key questions you can ask:
1. Tell me about your faith.
2. Do you attend church or other religious services?
3. If so, is this a help to you or is it a hindrance?

4. Does your faith influence the way you look at your illness and the way you think about your health?
5. What helps you most when you feel afraid or need help?
6. To whom can you turn for help?
7. Has God been of help to you in this illness? If so, how?
8. Do you know God personally? Is he in your life, your heart, your mind? How would you describe God?
9. Have you prayed about the illness or these problems?

These questions are open and non-threatening questions. They allow the sick person to talk about religion and faith if she so wishes, or to say simply that she prefers not to discuss it. In response to your inquiry about faith, many sick persons will describe their church membership. They may cite one or more of several benefits such as:
1. being with friends and getting support and help from them
2. learning more about God
3. finding joy and peace in worship
4. having opportunities to serve others

Affirm and reinforce the benefits they mention. You may now add that the church is about Jesus. He is the founder and the One we worship. What is of greatest benefit is having a personal relationship with Jesus. At the appropriate time, you can ask, "Have you ever invited Jesus himself to come into your heart and rule over your life?" If a person does not understand this question, but wants to know more about it, you can then explain simply the story of our faith. You will find this outlined in the following section.

With a person who has already expressed faith in Christ, you can discuss how Christ can be of help in coping with the illness or any of the problems mentioned.

With those who have not expressed any faith in Christ, or who are of another faith, and even with those who may seem resistant, you can simply say: "I am a Christian. In my Christian faith I have found resources that have been of help to me when I have been ill, or in dealing with problems similar to these you have mentioned. Would you like me to share what I have found that has been helpful?" If the person says yes, you are free to share. If the person says no, then move on to something else.

With a person of another faith or religious group, ask him to describe his faith to you. Be sure to listen with much interest. Even if you do not feel comfortable with that faith, demonstrate your interest *in the person* by listening openly, carefully, and with no negative expressions or reactions whatsoever. In this way, you keep open the relationship and the possibility of being of help to him. When you have listened to his story, you can now ask if he would like to hear your story.

In telling your story, be brief and stick to the essentials. Do not emphasize comparisons or contrasts with his faith story, but be ready to discuss them if he picks up on them. Avoid discussions or arguments about different religions, churches, denominations, or doctrines. These have no place in the clinic, and often lead to conflicts and negative emotions. Keep in mind at all times that our basic goal is to help persons get well. Faith, and especially faith in Christ, is helpful in this, but religious issues may not be. So avoid discussions about religious preferences or creeds.

Recommendations about church attendance

With those who ask to what church you belong, say simply that you belong to a church. You may want to indicate which one, if it seems appropriate. It would be good to add, "Here we are talking about faith, not church. Faith basically means a relationship with God, and that is what I have found to be important."

However, it is good for Christians to attend church and to be part of a spiritually alive body of believers. When a sick person comes into a personal relationship with Christ, or renews that relationship, encourage him or her to become an active part of a church fellowship. First of all, inquire about the church preference, and if he or she is comfortable with that church. If so, encourage the person to be active in the life of the church.

If a sick person has had no experience with church or does not now have a satisfactory church but seems to want to begin attending a church, you can invite her to go along with you to your church. In this way, you will be able to initiate her into church attendance and make her feel at ease in a worship service and church fellowship. Once she feels comfortable, you can suggest she may prefer to try another church in order to determine where she feels most comfortable.

The goal of this ministry is not to increase the membership of a particular church. However, part of the healing process is restoration to full life in the community, and becoming part of a church fellowship is helpful to all who have recently become Christian or have renewed their faith. Therefore, do whatever seems appropriate to make it easy for an unchurched person to become a part of a Christian fellowship.

Helping a Person Become a Christian

The greatest privilege we have as Christians is that of helping another person become a Christian, come into the Kingdom of God, and enter into eternal life. In reality, when a person establishes a personal relationship with Jesus, this has therapeutic benefits.

1. It gives a person hope for eternity, the "living hope" Peter describes in I Peter 1:3, 4. Hope itself has physiological benefits, for it enables our organ systems including the immune system to function better.
2. It provides joy and a new meaning and purpose for living. This also strengthens the body.
3. It makes available to a person the resources Christ has given us for coping better with stress, for restoring broken relationships, and for resolving fear, anxiety, and the many other negative feelings and thoughts that depress our organs and immune system.

As you discuss matters of faith with a sick person and find he does not have a relationship with Christ *but would like to have one*, then you can proceed with a simple explanation of how to become a Christian.

First, tell the story of our faith. It is important to remember that a person needs to hear the **whole story** and that the story begins at the beginning, namely, in Genesis:
- Who God is
- What the world is like
- Who we are
- What sin is and what it has done to us

Helping Hurting People

Only as a person understands the beginning of the story will he be able to comprehend fully the meaning and reason for salvation.

Here is a brief outline of the "whole story" that you can share quickly but carefully with a person.
1. God created the world. He made us as men and women. Everything God made is good including nature and humankind.
2. God loves us, knows each one of us by name, and wants us to love him, trust him, and obey the laws and instructions he has given us. He has given us these laws for our benefit, and those benefits include health and strength.
3. However, we have much pride in our hearts and we do not want to obey God. We want to follow our own desires, and so we refuse God and thus sin against him just as our ancestors Adam and Eve did.
4. Sin is very serious. It separates us from God and we die spiritually. Sin also causes much disorder between people, and can even make us sick. Because sin is serious and leads to death, either we die because of our sin or else someone else must die in our place.
5. God still loves us. He does not want us to die in our sin, and he wants us to come back to fellowship with him. So he came to us, as a man, to live among us. This man is Jesus Christ. We call him the Son of God because he is indeed God living as a man.
6. Jesus did die in our place, on the cross, and so he has paid the penalty for our sin. Then Jesus came back to life by rising from death. If we believe in Jesus and ask him to come into our heart to save us from sin and help us obey him, he will do so. Then we will not die because of our sin, for he has already died for us.
7. When Jesus comes into our heart, he shows us how to live a good life and gives us the wisdom, courage, and power to be good and not do evil. He also can help us solve our problems and even find healing when we are ill.

If a person does want to ask Jesus to come into his heart, help him pray this prayer.
"Jesus, I realize that I am a sinner but that you died in my place. I ask you to come into my heart now and live with me. Please forgive me of my sin, and help me to live now as I should live. Help me to love you as you love me. Thank you."

When a person accepts Christ, he needs help in growing in his faith.
1. He will need a Bible and guidance about how to read and study it.
2. He will need instruction in the faith. Talk with him about the importance of being in a good church (see the section above) and perhaps in a Bible study group.
3. If possible, schedule him to come back so you can continue to care for him. Tell him stories from the Bible about God, about Jesus, and about how we are to live.
4. If he asks you questions you cannot answer, respond simply by saying you do not know the answer but will discuss it with others and try to find the answer.

Now you can help this person to ask Christ to help him resolve worries, anxieties, fear, or other negative emotions in his heart. Suggest that he describe these problems to Christ in prayer, release them to him, and ask the Lord to heal the anguish they have caused and replace it with his peace. He can also ask help from Christ in resolving any conflicts between him and others in his family or circle of friends and associates.

Taking a Spiritual History

We will now look together at the important matter of praying sick persons, but before we do that, reflect on these questions:

Questions for reflection
1. Many people believe they are Christian because they belong to a church. How can you help them understand what it means to be a follower of Jesus?

2. Outline the steps a person follows in order to become a follower of Jesus?

3. What crucial needs does a new believer in Jesus have?

4. How can you help the new believer with these needs? In other words, what follow-up is necessary?

5. What kinds of questions or messages must be avoided in talking with people about matters of faith?

Homework
Read lesson 14 on Praying with Sick Persons in *Helping Hurting People*

Lesson 14
Praying with Sick Persons

Prayer is entering consciously into a reciprocal relationship with God in order to cooperate with him in accomplishing his purposes. It is a real and active power passing between God, the intercessor, and the person or object for which prayer is being made.

<u>The persistent widow</u>- Luke 18 : 1 - 8
1. The nature of prayer
    - rebellion against injustice, against what should not be
    - a means through whom God can work
2. The practice of prayer
    - persistence due to the belief in the power of prayer
    - faith that the power of God can work through us to bring change
3. God can change circumstances but usually does so only when he can do so through us
4. The magnitude of the problem determines the amount and intensity of prayer needed to deal with it. The greater the injustice or evil, the greater must be the magnitude and the intensity of prayer

<u>The Cycle of Prayer</u> – Revelation 8 : 1 - 5
1. God is listening to hear us pray.
2. Our prayer is like incense ascending to the Throne of God
3. When the incense container is full and our prayers have gone to God, then his purifying power comes down to work in the world.

Some diseases respond quickly to prayer. This is especially true for acute infections. Other diseases require much more prayer. This includes many malignancies, chronic infections, and diseases of long duration.

Prayer is work, and it can be hard, even exhausting work. We need to pray with our mind, our soul, and our spirit.

<u>Mind</u>:
Our thoughts should be focused on the person and the particular disease or aspects of the illness. We should be specific in our prayer. This is why knowing about the person's illness, worries, concerns, and problems is important. We can pray for coronary arteries, for the liver or kidneys, for the white blood cells and antibodies. We can ask God to help the person with specific needs, like a good night's sleep, a better appetite, or freedom from pain. We are bringing these matters to God to consult with him about them.

<u>Soul</u>:

Our feelings and emotions need to be involved. We can express them to God: our worry, concern, even our anger. Consider the many different emotions expressed in the Psalms. "The fervent prayer of a righteous person is effective and powerful" James 5 : 16.

<u>Spirit</u>:

In real prayer, we enter into the presence of the Almighty God. We are doing business with him. We are offering ourselves to him as a means through which his power can flow into the one for whom we are praying. Prayer is not manipulation of God. There is no magical formula that will require God to act as we want him to. Rather, prayer is entering into the work that we believe God wants to do and may already be doing and working with God to accomplish his will. Prayer is also listening. On occasion, as we pray, God will impress on our spirit a message we need to hear and obey. As our relationship with God deepens, we will be increasingly able to discern which of the thoughts that come to us are from God himself.

<u>Praying "in the will of God"</u>
1. God wills our health: John 10:10; Psalm 91:14-16; Deuteronomy 28
2. Jeremiah 29:11-13: "For I know the plans I have for you," declares the Lord, "plans to prosper you and not to harm you, plans to give you hope and a future. Then you will call upon me and come to me and pray to me, and I will listen to you. You will seek me and find me when you seek me with all your heart."
3. Physical healing does not always come. Nevertheless, God is at work in our circumstances (illness) for our good – Romans 8:28. What good can come of it?
   a. peace, patience, and trust in God
   b. wisdom and more understanding of self, of life, and of God
4. Heart healing can come no matter how sick a person may be, for Christ can heal the heart of anyone.
5. Heart healing, with its consequent peace and joy, can strengthen the body and enable it to cope better with whatever the disease is. In other words, heart healing creates a favorable environment for the person in their struggle with the disease.
6. So we can ask God to heal this person "in his time, and according to his plan."

<u>Prayer should be specific</u>
1. We can pray about the disease and the affected organs.
2. We can pray about specific symptoms, that God will relieve them.
3. We can pray for the family and the personal life of the sick person.
4. We can pray for the caregivers and the various treatments.

<u>Bringing problems into the presence of the Lord</u>
1. When a person wants prayer and has specific problems, ask him or her to be quiet for a moment and focus their attention on the real concerns of the heart:
   - the disease, or symptoms
   - a particular worry, concern, or painful feeling
2. Now ask him to take these concerns, problems, or feelings and offer them to Jesus, placing them in his hands, and asking him to take them away.
3. Have him try to imagine Jesus doing this.

4. Now he can listen for any word the Lord may say. If the Lord does speak, the person may want to share it with you.
5. Then after a moment, pray audibly, bringing these concerns to the Lord yourself.

<u>Praying with an unconscious person</u>
1. Hearing is the last sense to disappear, so an unconscious person may hear what you are saying.
2. Therefore, NEVER talk negatively in the presence of an unconscious person.
3. Talk to the person by name as if she can hear you.
4. Speak a word of encouragement.
5. Share a portion of Scripture.
6. Pray for healing "according to God's will and in his time."

<u>Prayer speaks to three persons</u>
1. to God
2. to your own heart
3. to the mind and heart of the person with whom you pray. That person may hear a word you spoke in the prayer that brings peace, joy, or even healing to her heart.

<u>Always ask for permission before you pray</u>
1. This is essential for legal purposes as well as for good spiritual care.
2. Most sick persons will want you to pray.
3. If someone does not want you to do so, then don't insist on it.
4. If they do want prayer, ask if there are other problems or concerns they would like you to pray about. This can often uncover other related problems that need to be discussed and brought to the Lord for resolution.

<u>Why are some people not healed?</u>
Why does God heal some people and not others? Why does a 'miracle of healing' occur to someone who has cancer, but not to someone else? This question is not only difficult, but it may lead some people to lose their faith in God. 'God healed John. Why does he refuse to heal me?'

<u>Here are possible approaches to this question.</u>
1. God is sovereign. He heals those whom he chooses to heal but does not heal others for reasons we do not know. We know that God is indeed sovereign and we must accept that. However, there is a certain fatalism in this, and also a hint that it is God's fault that he is not healing me.
2. The second possibility is that certain factors, or obstacles, may be present that are preventing healing. Unless these factors are dealt with, God cannot make the healing happen. This means that the 'ball is in our court' and we must re-evaluate our situation to try to find what is blocking the healing. The danger here is in creating a false guilt that "it is my fault I am not being healed."
3. A third possibility is that, subconsciously, the person does not want to be healed.
4. The best option is recognizing that we do not know and probably cannot know but must simply trust in the goodness of God. At the same time, we make sure that we have dealt with any known obstacles to healing.

So let us look at some factors that could prevent healing.

A wrong diagnosis or incorrect treatment

I (DF) was once asked to pray for a lady in Indonesia who has been paralyzed from the waist down for two years. She had been examined in excellent hospitals, and that included a CT scan of her lower back and legs. No cause could be found, and she was referred for psychiatric help. She was under the care of a Christian neurologist, and he asked me to pray with the lady who was a Christian. Before we prayed, I noted that her hands also seemed to be weak and suggested further examinations. I then prayed for God to heal her and to give wisdom to the physicians who were caring for her. The following day, the neurologist ordered a CT scan of the spine of her neck. This revealed a tumor pressing on the spinal cord in her neck. The tumor, which was benign, was removed a few days later, with complete recovery from all her paralysis. God did answer our prayer for healing by giving wisdom to those who cared for her to lead them to the right diagnosis.

Personal unconfessed sin

If we hold onto sin in our life – wrong actions or sinful attitudes – this can keep God from accomplishing his purpose in us. We read about this in Isaiah 59: 1-2, and also in Mark 11: 25. In the book *God, Medicine, and Miracles*, I (DF) describe how my sinful abuse of my body through overwork kept God from healing my chronic liver disease. Painful relationships producing hostility and anger, with the refusal to forgive someone who has wronged us, can indeed be an obstacle to God's power to heal us. Here is where the exercise of doing a life review can be helpful. We come to this in lesson 15.

Lack of faith

Jesus speaks about this in Mark 11 : 22 - 24. We need to understand what Jesus means by this, for misunderstanding this can lead to much error. It is not our faith that heals us. Rather it is the power of Jesus that heals us. By faith, Jesus means that it is our faith that brings us to Jesus in the confidence that he can heal us, for he is the healer. But if we fail to come to Jesus and to ask for his healing, he can do nothing.

We see a good example of this in Mark 5 with the woman who was bleeding. Her faith led her to touch the tassel on Jesus' robe in the confidence she would be healed, and she was. We see it also in Mark 2 : 1 - 12 in the story of the four men who brought their paralyzed friend to Jesus. When Jesus saw the faith of *these four men*, he then proceeded to heal the sick man. The faith of the men did not heal their friend; Jesus healed him. But it was their faith that motivated them to *bring their friend to Jesus.*

A mystery

We also must recognize that what we consider to be good, in this case physical healing, may not be what God considers to be best for us. He may have a purpose for us that he is accomplishing in us using the illness or suffering. This was the situation of Job. He did not know, until the end, that his great suffering had a divine purpose to show to others, and especially to the enemy of our souls, that the faith of a man can triumph in spite of extremely difficult circumstances. So our faith must be such that we trust God to work in us what he knows is best even though it may not appear to us to be good.

<u>We need to consider all of these possibilities and work through each one.</u>
1. God is sovereign. If we come to him in faith that he will work his good plan in us, we can have the peace that he will indeed do this.
2. We can encourage the medical caregivers to examine every possibility, and pray that God will give them wisdom to do so.
3. We can encourage the sick person to do a self-examination, alone or with the help of a wise and trusted counselor, to see if any obstacles to healing exist, either in feelings that need to be changed, unconfessed sins that need to be brought to God, painful relationships that require forgiveness and healing, or behavior that is unhealthy. However, we must NEVER say to a sick person who has not been physically healed: "You must still have some unconfessed sin or another obstacle in your life." Only the sick person can determine that. We cannot.
4. We all must realize that much mystery remains in the area of illness and healing. In spite of increasing scientific and psychological understanding, there is still much we do not yet know and must therefore commit into the hands of a God whom we trust and who is the God of love.

Helping Hurting People

Questions for reflection
1. Share with the group, or write out for yourself, experiences where, in spite of much prayer, physical healing did not occur. In retrospect, why do you think this was so?

2. Share other experiences where you saw answers to prayer. Why was this so?

3. How can you respond to someone who asks why God is not answering his (her) prayers for healing?

4. How can our effectiveness in prayer increase?

Homework
1. Read *God, Medicine, and Miracles*, pages 198 – 201
2. Read lesson 15 on Doing a Life Review in *Helping Hurting People*

Lesson 15
Doing a Life Review
See GMM, pages 198 – 201

Principles:
1. *What happens at any point in life influences all of subsequent development.*
2. *The present is the sum of all that has happened in the past.*

During an illness, looking back at our past, from childhood to the present, can be helpful if done carefully and prayerfully. Painful memories, unresolved conflicts, and hurting feelings can be examined and dealt with. The perspective of King David as outlined in Psalm 139 is very helpful. He knew that his whole life, from conception to the present, was known to God, and he finished his review by exclaiming, "Search me, O God, and know my heart. Try me and know my anxieties. And see if there is any wicked way in me, and lead me in the way everlasting." Verses 23 and 24. 'In the way everlasting' really means 'in the way of health, now and for eternity.'

A symbol

Here is a symbol of our life that is useful in envisaging where we are now. Life is like a river with a beginning, a winding trajectory, and a gradually increasing current and volume as other streams come into it. Remember in our discussion of the story in Exodus 15 that water is a symbol of our inner life, our spirit. So the water in this symbolic river signifies our inner life.
1. A river begins at its source. The source receives water from under the ground.
2. A tiny stream comes out of the source and begins flowing downhill.
3. The stream twists and turns, going around rocks, hills, and any obstacles in its way.
4. At certain places the stream flows rapidly. There may be rapids, even waterfalls.
5. At other places the flow is smooth and the water is placid.
6. Other little streams come into it, bringing water from different areas.
    - Some of this water may be clear.
    - Water from other streams may be muddy, contaminated, or polluted.
7. All water coming into the stream mingles with the water in the stream.
8. Eventually the stream becomes a small river, and it continues to deepen and widen.
9. Bigger tributaries join it, each one bringing different water into the main stream.
10. The water in the river at any given point is the sum of all of the water that has come from the original stream and all the tributaries.

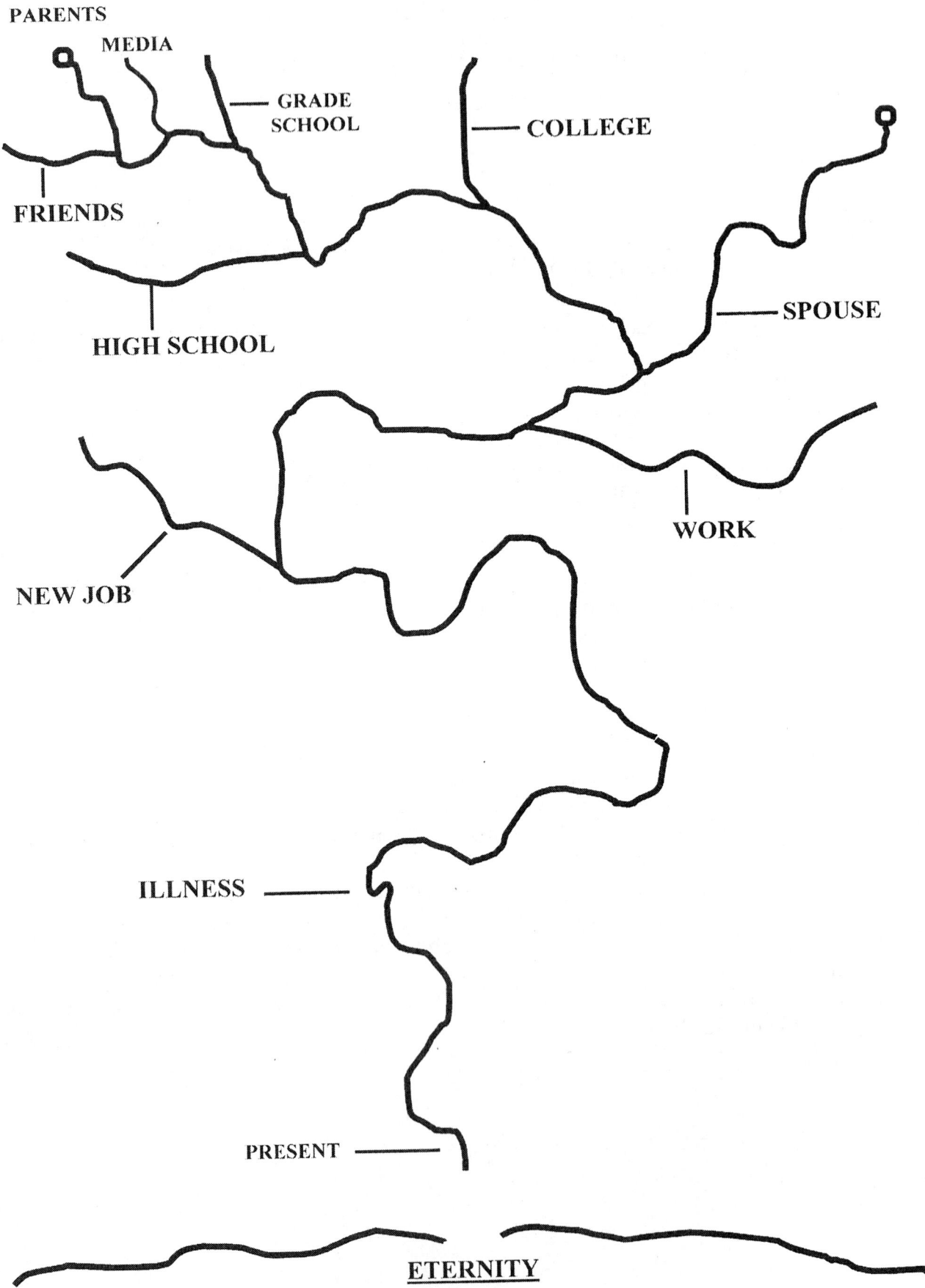

Doing a Life Review

How is life like a river?

Source
1. Our parents, biological or sociological, with their beliefs, values, and life style
2. Our genetic heritage
3. Our cultural heritage, the collective beliefs and values of our group

Influences in early life
1. Parents, siblings, other relatives
2. Events
   - Happy, pleasant, constructive surroundings and events
   - Traumatic, unpleasant, or evil circumstances or surroundings
3. Media, a powerful influence that continues throughout life
4. Culture

Many tributaries
1. Early childhood playmates
2. School: new ideas and experiences
3. Church, community, wider circle of friends
4. Peers
5. The media, the internet, etc.
6. Further education, military service
7. Employment – challenges, opportunities, new associates, with good or bad influences
8. Marriage – a major tributary
9. Major events – success, advancement, a new home
10. Disasters – accidents, displacements, war, loss of a loved one, serious illnesses

Doing a life review

In order for you to help others with this, it is beneficial to go through this exercise yourself. If you can afford to take one or more days to do this – a personal retreat – you will find it helpful. Take a big sheet of paper, newsprint for example. Using your imagination, begin to draw the 'river' of your life with its many twists and curves. Then go back to the beginning and draw in the many tributaries that have contributed to your life. You may want to use crayons of different colors for this. Blue might represent clear water, green being positive influences. Brown, orange, or red might indicate negative or harmful influences. Give rein to your imagination and let your creative juices flow in depicting your life. How much of the brown, orange or red water is still in your mainstream now?

1. This takes time. Do it thoughtfully and carefully.
2. Study Psalm 139. At every point, pray verses 23 and 24.
3. Note down the many good influences that have affected your life. Make a list of them on a separate sheet(s) of paper, or in a notebook. Thank God for them. Can any of these good influences help you now? Read Psalm 143 : 5 and 6
4. Try to identify one by one:
   - Bad influences that have "muddied up the water of your spirit"
   - Traumatic events: disasters, abuses, and how you handled them
   - Obstacles to maturity and spiritual development and how you handled them
   - Pollutants that have contaminated the "water" of your spirit
   - Write these also in another notebook or on separate sheets of paper so you can come back to them.

Helping Hurting People

<u>Obstacles to maturity, or pollutants, that can have long-term harmful effects</u>
1. Heritage
   - Generational problems: physical diseases, unhealthy behaviors like substance abuse or compulsive behaviors, unhealthy attitudes
   - Parental traits: strong emotions, bad attitudes, unhealthy relationships, focus on materialism
2. Early childhood environment
   - Emotional starvation
   - Abuse: emotional, physical, sexual
3. Bad choices
   - Of companions who brought in evil influences
   - Unhealthy or destructive behaviors
   - Sin: knowing what is right, yet doing wrong
4. Traumatic events
   - Parental divorce, breakdown of one's own marriage
   - Failure at school or at work, with loss of self-esteem
   - Serious family problems
   - Other disasters
5. Unhealthy attitudes of your own: anger, temper tantrums, fear, phobias, anxiety

<u>How to deal with the negative or harmful influences, obstacles, or events of the past</u>
1. Do you feel there is still a negative influence now because of certain things? Do past memories still bring pain, fear, or emotional problems you would like to get rid of?
2. Can you reflect on a negative or harmful past influence without becoming upset or depressed?
   - If so, describe it carefully to yourself, and then to the Lord.
   - It is often helpful to write this description on paper.
   - Then in prayer give it to the Lord.
   - Ask him to purify the harmful influences, remove the inner pain coming from them, and replace the painful feelings with his peace.
   - Then tear up or burn what you have written and tell your heart it is gone.
   - Scientific research shows that when people write down painful or disturbing circumstances in their life, the immune system actually becomes stronger.
3. If a past memory is too painful or depressing yet you still feel you must deal with it:
   - Ask God to show you to whom you can go for help, wise counsel, prayer, and support.
   - With the help of that person, bring the problem to the Lord for healing.
4. Once you have given the past problem to the Lord, do not keep reflecting on it. When the memory does return, simply remind yourself that the Lord has taken away the evil effects and healed your spirit.

<u>Remember: There is a Healer.</u>
1. There is a Balm in Gilead to make the wounded whole. Jeremiah 8:22
2. By his wounds we have been healed. I Peter 2:24
3. Rejoice in the Lord always, again I say rejoice. Phil. 4:4

Results of a life review
1. "Purifying the water" of your spirit will make you and your body stronger and better able to cope with whatever problems or illnesses do occur.
2. This does not "guarantee" health or healing, but it does promote them.
3. When you do this and then live daily in an open relationship with the Lord, you can trust him to help you handle all that comes. You no longer need to worry because the Lord is a better "worrier" than you are.

Helping another person do this
When a person you are helping seems to have one or more serious issues to deal with, this exercise may be helpful. Explain how reflecting on past events, even back to childhood, can be useful. Show her the picture of the river and explain how this is a symbol of our life. You can perhaps share how you have used this symbol to reflect on your own life and how it has benefited you.

If she seems interested in doing this, go through the steps outlined here. Show her Psalm 139 and encourage her to ask for God's help in doing this. Emphasize taking time to do this when there will be no distractions. Explain also that it is by no means simply an effort to find the bad things. She must look for the many good things that have happened, write them down, give thanks for them, and take delight in them.

The personal inventory may bring up one or more specific areas that need resolution or healing:
1. A painful memory of trauma, abuse, or a bad decision
2. Anger against a parent, a spouse, a sibling, a child, or someone else
3. Compulsive thoughts, fantasies, or behavior such as internet pornography
4. Particular fears or disturbing phobias

Some of these situations can be deep, complex, and difficult to deal with. They may require the help of someone trained professionally in that area of concern. On the other hand, a deep encounter with Jesus may cut through to the core of the anxiety or pain, resolve it, and restore peace. Here is how you can try to help the person bring the burden or painful area to Jesus in a prayerful, not threatening, and often healing manner.

The person should describe the painful issue as clearly as possible, either by taking time to write out a description of it, or by telling it to you as a safe and trustworthy listener. When she has done this, ask her if she would like to release this concern to Jesus, to place it in his hands, and to ask him to remove it. If she is willing, one of the following symbolic acts can be helpful.

If she has written out her painful story, suggest that she take a red pen or marker and draw a cross over the written account. Then in prayer, she can give this story to Jesus, reminding herself that Jesus died on the cross to take away sin and evil from us and to purify us from all our wrongdoing. She can now tear the page or pages into shreds and throw them in the wastebasket. Or, if circumstances permit, she can set fire to the page(s) and watch the story burn up. Give her the verse in I Peter 5:7 – "Cast all your cares on him, for he cares for you." This is the assurance that the problem is gone. Now pray with her asking Jesus to heal the pain of the problem and replace the pain with his peace.

Another helpful act can be, after writing out the story, to fold it, put it into an envelope, and tie the envelope to the string of a helium balloon. Then go outdoors and release the balloon. This says a powerful word to the heart of the person – "It's gone!"

These symbolic acts are a word spoken to the heart that the problem is now in Jesus' hands and he has removed it. It is gone, and he has replaced it with his peace. The memory of whatever it was may return but the pain of it should be gone. Counsel her that if the memory of the situation does return, she should not dwell on it but should quickly remind herself that Jesus has taken care of the problem.

Ask her to come back to see you within a week. It is very important for you to monitor how well she is handling this exercise, or if it is too much for her. She can describe how this is going, what she has been able to accomplish, and if there are really difficult places she cannot deal with. You also can look for signs of anxiety or depression and evaluate how serious they are. If she seems to be having real difficulty in handling this, discuss with her the advisability of seeking a professionally trained person to help her with these areas. Suggest that she discuss this with her physician, or ask if she would like you to do this for her.

Some people object that we should not dwell on the past. This is not dwelling on the past but is rather "cleaning up" the past. Some quote the Apostle Paul who said he tried to forget the past and to keep striving to reach what is ahead (Philippians 3 : 13). The reality is that we cannot truly forget the past until we have dealt with it. Paul himself did this, and he described it in Romans chapter 7 and also in Philippians 3 : 1 – 11.

Finding Happiness, Satisfaction, and Purpose for Life

Here is another useful tool to help people who are facing limitations imposed on them by illness or the aging process. In fact, this can also help anyone who is not satisfied with his life situation, or who is striving to grow emotionally and spiritually. From ancient times philosophers have taught that we, as human beings, find happiness, satisfaction, meaning, and purpose in life on four levels of life.

Level one

This is the level of sense experience, of what is pleasing to our sight, hearing, touch, or feeling. It may be a delicious meal, a beautiful sunset, a moving piece of music, or any other pleasurable experience. God created us with five senses so that we can enjoy the physical world in which we live.

Level two

This is the level of ego gratification, of that which makes us feel good about ourselves. Honor, prestige, affirmation, promotion, and encouragement all can give happiness and satisfaction.

Level three

On this level we move out toward other people, and find happiness in service, in helping others, and in healthy relationships with others.

Level four

This is the spiritual level, where we find happiness, satisfaction, and purpose in a relationship with God and with the spiritual dimension of life. The mature person has a harmonious balance between all of these levels, and is able to find satisfaction on all four levels. When conflicts between the levels occur, he or she can make satisfactory decisions and adaptations in order to maintain inner harmony.

The Bible affirms this concept. In Matthew 6 : 33, Jesus says, "Seek first the Kingdom of God (*level four*) and his righteousness (*level three*) and all these others things (*levels two and one*) will be given to you." The Bible instructs us on the priorities we should have in investing our time and energy on the different levels.

When people face serious illness, or when the aging process has progressed fairly far, physical limitations increase, and the possibilities for honor, prestige, etc. diminish. People who have found happiness and purpose primarily on levels one and two, aging and/or serious illness become serious threats to them. In this case, we can help them by encouraging them to refocus their remaining time and energy on levels three and four.

Most people, even with serious physical limitations, can reach out to other people (telephone, writing, visiting), relate to them, and be of help to them. Almost everyone can invest more in a relationship with God through prayer, faith, and reading God's Word and reflecting on it. By enabling such people to shift their desires from what is becoming unattainable to what is still attainable and can be fulfilling for the present and also for eternity, we can enable them to cope with even immense threats to their well-being.

FOUR LEVELS OF MEANING

- SPIRITUAL
- RELATIONSHIPS
- EGO GRATIFICATION
- SENSUAL

Doing a Life Review

Helping people find meaning and fulfillment in life

How can we help sick persons with this? The best way to start is to apply this to yourself. Take an hour or so of undistracted time and reflect on how you find happiness and purpose in your own life.
1. What things make you really happy? – things you especially like to do?
2. What do you enjoy doing on a day off? Or on vacation?
3. What would you like to have happen in your life now?
4. What things make you really feel good? Important? Happy about yourself? Appreciated?
5. Who are the important people in your life, and how well do you get along with them? What do you enjoy doing with other people?
6. What support groups do you have that help you?
7. Do you find pleasure serving other people in need? How do you do this?
8. Where does God fit into your life? Do you spend fulfilling time thinking about him, praying to him, studying about him?
9. Are there other spiritual activities you enjoy?
10. When you want to do something on one level but an urgent matter comes up on another level, how do you handle this conflict in priorities?

Many people are depressed or suffer from a low self-image. As you establish a caring relationship with such a person, explain these four areas of life in which we can find identity, meaning, and fulfillment. Go through the description given here and show them the diagram of the four levels. When you feel the person has understood this, ask him how he would evaluate his own current situation in the light of this.

This may be difficult for some people to do, for it is rather abstract. Try to give concrete examples of how you find happiness on each of these levels. For those facing increasing limitations in their life, ask one or more of the following questions:
1. Are there things you like to do that you can no longer do?
2. Are there other things you like and can still do?
3. Can you make new friends? Or talk more frequently with old friends? Or be of service to others?
4. Can you find increased happiness in your relationship with God?
    a. prayer and meditation
    b. bible reading
    c. listening to hymns or other music
5. What support groups do you have that help you?
    a. family
    b. church
    c. groups of friends
    d. of others

If a person has no such support network, what can you and your church, or other churches, do to provide a support group for that person? NO ONE SHOULD FEEL ABANDONED.

Helping Hurting People

Questions for reflection
1. Write a brief paragraph about how you can describe to a person struggling with a chronic illness the benefits of a life review and how he or she can do it.

2. How can you explain to a sick person the way in which painful experiences even in early childhood can still affect life and health in adulthood?

3. How can we help someone who has a debilitating or disfiguring illness find new purpose and meaning for life?

4. How can you help an older person whose physical and social abilities are diminishing to find happiness during the remaining years?

Personal recommendation
5. Begin to do this life review yourself. Start with your heritage and early childhood and see what you come up with. Use a notebook to record your reflections and feelings.

6. How do you sort out priorities between your levels of meaning and happiness when conflicts arise between demands on the different levels? For example, an urgent family need occurs just before a planned vacation.

Homework
Read lesson 16 on Self-Identity in *Helping Hurting People*

Lesson 16
A Problem of Self-Identity

Self-identity, or self-understanding or self-esteem, is at the center of our personality. It is our answer to the basic question of life: "Who am I?" Our self-understanding affects our life style, behavior, and health. An inadequate or painful self-identity can lead to problems of depression, eating disorders, acting out, compulsive behaviors, and even a diminished or disordered immune system. It therefore is a crucial health issue.

Self-identity is shaped very early in life. Experiences in babyhood and early childhood have a great influence on our understanding of who we are as persons. Self-understanding can and does change during adult years, but is usually more difficult. It can be radically altered, however, by life-changing experiences.

Some causes of low self-esteem
Many factors can give a person a poor or painful self-understanding.
1. A dysfunctional family
2. Rejection by one or both parents
3. The absence of one or both parents
4. Gender rejection: "You are a girl, but we wanted a boy." This can lead to a woman believing she is no good because she is a woman.
5. Constantly being told: "You are no good. You will never amount to anything."
6. Ethnic or cultural background not well accepted
7. Low economic or social status of the family
8. Early childhood fright, from illness, trauma, external violence or the impact of media violence. Such experiences, even at birth or in the first few days of life, can engrave panic or a death image deep in the inaccessible memories. Yet this can have a powerful influence on dreams, feelings, and behavior throughout life.

Identity problems go very deep in the personality and may require in-depth professional Christ-centered counseling. On the other hand, a spiritually sensitive spiritual caregiver can often be helpful in bringing such a problem to the surface and, on occasion, can help a person find a new positive self-identity through Christ.

One or more simple questions may open this area for fruitful discussion.
1. How do you feel about yourself?
2. Do you feel good about who you are?
3. Do you ever wish you had been born as someone else?
4. Has someone ever told you that you are worthless, or will never amount to anything?

How can we help a person with low self-esteem?
With a person who has a low self-image, we can ask about the circumstances leading to that. We can inquire about early childhood and family issues. A warm, affirming, and functional family are of great benefit in enabling a young person to develop a satisfactory self image. The converse can lead to deep problems with self esteem. Dysfunctional or abusive parents often distort the self-image of a child or young person and make emotional maturity more difficult.

A low self-image may be associated with a poor image of God, who he is and what he is like. Our image of God is strongly influenced by the image we have of our earthly father. Many people have a poor or even traumatic image of their father and so cannot relate to God as their heavenly Father. We must help them deal with this, often before we can help with their own self-image.

Genesis and self-image

In the book of Genesis we learn much about God and also about ourselves. God is good, totally faithful and trustworthy, and is full of sacrificial love. Other passages, especially in the Psalms and also in the New Testament, help us see the real nature of God as good, as love, and as the One who cares for us, nourishes us, protects us, leads and guides us. Helping a person understand the marvelous nature of God as a truly loving Father can do wonders in the deep psyche.

Genesis explains clearly that God, who is good, who is love, and who is faithful, has put his image into our hearts and we are to try to become like him. He has put his image into both men and women, and they are equal in God's sight and should be considered equal in the sight of one another. The Bible gives no credence to male domination or to female inferiority. Many passages in Scripture indicate the feminine or maternal aspects of God. This makes clear that femininity is equal to masculinity in God's sight because both have come from him.

If it seems appropriate, suggest to such a person that he or she study the book of Genesis with the purpose of seeing who God is, what he is like, and what is his relationship with us whom he has created. A similar study of the Psalms can also be helpful. The person can also examine the early chapters of Genesis to discover who we are as persons, the responsibilities God has given us, and what our relationship should be with him.

Many passages in Scripture make clear our identity as children of God once we come into a personal relationship with God through Christ. This is why a clear explanation of what it means to have a relationship with Christ is so important and why we can invite, although never pressure, a person to make that major step. Here follows a list of some key passages that indicate our new identity in Christ. When a person has asked Christ into his or her heart, suggest memorizing these verses and referring to them whenever thoughts of poor self-esteem or self accusation recur.

- I am a child of God – John 1:12
- I am a friend of Jesus – John 15:15
- I am the temple of God – 1Cor. 6:19
- I resemble God – Genesis 1:27
- God wants me to be like him – Ephesians 5 : 1
- God loves me – 1 Thessalonians 1:4
- Jesus died for me even though I am a sinner because he loves me
  John 3 : 16, I Peter 3 : 18; I John 3 : 16

A helpful book on self image for those who are want to explore their relationship with God is *A New Identity in Christ* by Neil Anderson, Regal Books, Ventura, CA

A Problem of Self-Identity

Questions for reflection
1. How did Dr. Sherry figure out the real problems of James? (told on the DVD)

2. What steps did she follow in helping him find new meaning for his life?

3. What prevented Pastor John from being a successful pastor? (told on the DVD)

4. How did his colleagues help restore his self image?

5. What does this story demonstrate about the power of words?

6. How can we help our own children develop a healthy self-image?

Homework
Read lesson 17 on Anger, Illness, and Forgiving Others in *Helping Hurting People*

Lesson 17
Anger, Illness, and Forgiving Others
God, Medicine, and Miracles, *chapter 10*

Anger: What should we do with it?
　We have discussed anger, a very powerful emotion that can quickly provoke us into action. We have likewise talked about how chronic anger, anger that is retained and often suppressed down into the deep recesses of the heart can, over time, damage tissues and organs and lead to chronic illness. What makes us angry? Why do we like to hold onto our anger?

There are two general causes for anger:
1. When someone says or does something that threatens us, we get angry. When someone hurts us, we get angry. Anger is a protective emotion. It stimulates the production of adrenalin that prepares us for actions to protect ourselves.
2. When we see someone doing something to other people that harms them, we also often get angry. We get angry when we see violence hurting or destroying people. I get angry at cancer or at AIDS because these diseases destroy life.

　Once again we can look at the example of Jesus. He got angry, but he handled his anger properly. He controlled his anger; he did not allow it to control him. He then used the energy of his anger to accomplish good things. In chapter eleven of Mark's gospel we see the account of Jesus' entrance into the Temple in Jerusalem. He saw the evil which many religious leaders were doing to others, exploiting them through price gouging. He did not react immediately but, as Mark says, he "looked around on everything, and since it was late, he went out of the Temple and back to Bethany." I believe this was deliberate anger control. He spent the night, got his emotional energy under control, carefully planned what his response would be to the evil inflicted on others by unrighteous people, and the next day he went into action.

　How are we to handle anger when it comes? The Apostle Paul gives us marvelous psychologically sound counsel in Ephesians 4 : 26 and 27. He says:
　When you become angry, do not let your anger lead you into sin.
　Do not let the sun go down on your anger.
　Don't give the devil an opportunity.

Here is what Paul is saying:
1. Anger is a normal emotion, and it is morally neutral. It comes to all of us. We are made in God's image. God becomes angry, and so do we.
2. Anger is a powerful emotion, yet we are to control it, and not let it control us.
3. When something occurs that stimulates anger in us, we must take care of the matter quickly – "before the sun goes down." We must take care both of the anger itself and work through whatever the circumstance is that has provoked us to anger. In other words, don't hold onto anger. Don't stuff it down inside and suppress it into some obscure region of the heart.

4. If we do hold onto anger or stuff it down inside, it gives the devil an opportunity. An opportunity for what? For us to become ill.

If we take this counsel seriously and apply it whenever circumstances occur that provoke anger, we will be psychologically and spiritually healthy. Otherwise, the anger will lead us into resentment and bitterness. Bitterness poisons the spirit which, in turn, can produce illness of the body. There is growing evidence that deeply buried anger can damage certain collagen tissues and lead to rheumatoid arthritis. It can upset the immune system and lead to an auto-immune disease. It can suppress the immune system, opening the door to chronic infections.

How can we resolve anger?

Life is full of hurts, hurts that we cause to each other. We bump into each other, wound each other with sharp words, and disrupt or fracture relationships. All of this brings much pain into our hearts.

Forgiveness is the means God has provided for us to mend relationships and to heal the pain and anguish of these hurts. To quote Lewis Smedes: "Forgiveness is God's invention for coming to terms with a world in which, despite their best intentions, people are unfair to each other and hurt each other deeply. God began by forgiving us. He invites us to forgive each other."

Forgiveness of others is God's way for us to deal with the hurts we feel we do not deserve. It is difficult for us to forgive others because it goes against the grain of our pride. We enjoy condemning the offender in our heart, for it is a boost to our own ego. So forgiving others requires an *act of the will* that overrides our feelings and desires.

What happens when someone offends us?
1. We hurt. It is painful, upsetting, and threatening.
2. We become angry, and can even develop hatred toward the offender.
3. We condemn the offender in our heart, often before God, and sometimes before others. At the same time we justify ourselves: "HE did this to ME!"
4. We plan revenge.
5. We become filled with resentment, bitterness and anger. These feelings can cause psychological and even physical suffering and illness.
6. We must then make a decision: Does my enjoyment of the resentment and condemnation of the offender outweigh the pain of my bitterness? If I decide it does not, I can then release my condemnation of the offender by forgiving him.
7. When I do forgive, I am released and healed of the pain of my bitterness.

Why should I forgive someone who has offended me?
1. God requires it: Matthew 6:12-15; Mark 11:24-25; Ephesians 4:32; Colossians 3:13
2. Revenge is not a viable alternative, for it leads to escalating mutual offenses.
3. I am set free from the inner garbage I have accumulated because of the offense. In other words, it is in my own best interest to forgive the offender.
4. I can then reestablish relationships of harmony and respect.
5. I can, and must, forgive someone even if he does not apologize or is unavailable. Jesus did this on the cross. Stephen forgave his executioners.

Jesus told a remarkable parable about forgiveness. It is in Matthew 18 : 21 – 35.
Then Peter came to Jesus and asked, "Lord, if my brother keeps on sinning against me, how many times do I have forgive him? Seven times?"

"No, not seven times," answered Jesus, "but seventy times seven, because the kingdom of heaven is like this. Once there was a king who decided to check on the servants' accounts. He had just begun to do so when one of them was brought in who owed him millions of dollars. The servant did not have enough money to pay his debt, so the king ordered him to be sold as a slave, with his wife and his children and all that he had, in order to pay off his debts. The servant fell on his knees before the king. "Be patient with me," he begged, "and I will pay you everything!" The king felt sorry for him and so he forgave him the debt and let him go.

Then the man went out and met one of his fellow servants who owed him a few dollars. He grabbed him and started choking him. "Pay back what you owe me!" he said. His fellow servant fell down and begged him, "Be patient with me, and I will pay you back!" But he refused; instead, he had him thrown into jail until he should pay back the debt.

When the other servants saw what had happened, they were very upset and went to the king and told him everything. So he called the servant in. "You worthless servant," he said. "I forgave you the whole amount you owed me, just because you asked me to. You should have had mercy on your fellow servant, just as I had mercy on you." The king was very angry and he sent the servant to jail until he should pay back the whole amount. And Jesus concluded, "This is how my Father in heaven will treat every one of you unless you forgive your brother from your heart."

Many people who come to you for help will tell you a story of having been hurt by someone, usually a close family member: divorce, deception, an insult, or an unresolved conflict. The anger, bitterness, and resentment – the 'grudge' – against the offender is affecting their health and may even be causing some of their symptoms. This is the 'prison' into which people shut themselves when they harbor a grudge or hold onto bitterness and anger. Scientific research is now demonstrating how the act of forgiving an offender can relieve physical pain, strengthen the immune system, and even restore health. Research shows an inverse relationship between our level of hostility and the strength of the immune system. You will have the privilege of helping many to understand forgiveness, decide to forgive their offender, and thus find release, restoration of inner peace, and improved health.

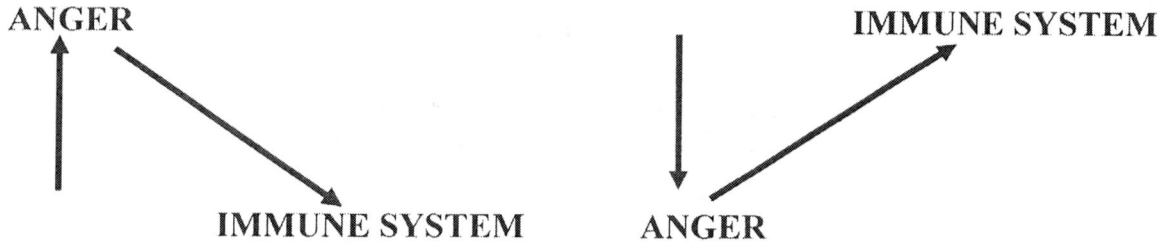

<u>What is forgiveness?</u>
1. Forgiveness does not mean condoning or excusing the wrong.
2. When I forgive someone, I turn him over to God. I agree before God to stop judging and condemning him, and I recognize God as the only righteous Judge. The other person may be as wrong as wrong can be, but I will no longer be his judge. I release him to God, letting go of my judgment and letting God be his sole judge.

3. I then ask Christ to purify my heart of the anger, resentment, and bitterness I have held, to heal these wounds by his blood, and to let his peace fill my heart.

<u>Here is something quite remarkable:</u> - When we forgive, it blesses the one forgiven
Think back to a time when you wronged someone else and that person forgave you. Perhaps it was a parent, a sibling, or a close friend. Was that forgiveness a real gift to you? How did it make you fell – grateful? - relieved? - released from guilt and shame? Did it open the way for reconciliation to occur?

Perhaps someone has offended you. Can you offer that person the gift of forgiveness? At first sight this seems ridiculous. How can I give a gift to someone who has hurt me? But remember that Jesus did precisely that on the cross. He also told us to love our enemies and bless those who hurt us.

Here are some helpful steps that can enable you to offer the gift of forgiveness to someone who has willfully hurt you.
1. Think about the offender and why he may have hurt you. Try to empathize with him. Was he himself hurting and perhaps reaching out awkwardly for help?
2. Think again about what happened. What really hurt you? Try to look at it as objectively as possible.
3. Make a decision to forgive. In forgiving the offender, you are releasing your condemnation and your anger to God and asking him to bless and hopefully change the offender.
4. Once you have done that, it is done. You may continue to remember the offense, but that is normal. You can simply remind yourself that forgiveness has been granted and that all condemnation and anger are finished.

My forgiving the offender can enable God to work more effectively in the life of the offender. Jesus told his disciples: "Whatever you bind on earth will be bound in heaven, and whatever you loose on earth will be loosed in heaven" (Matthew 16:19). This is serious and we need to understand this principle. If I refuse to forgive someone who has offended me, I am binding that person spiritually, and this can impede the work that God (in heaven) wants to do in him. I am in effect standing between the offender and the Holy Spirit, blocking the Spirit's convicting power in the life of the offender. On the other hand, when I forgive the offender, I remove those bonds and thus loose the person. God's Spirit is now able to work more freely and effectively in that person.

When Stephen cried, "Father, lay not this sin to their charge," the young man Saul heard him say that (Acts chapter 7). That statement might have played a role in Saul's subsequent conversion.

<u>Here is another important principle</u>
The refusal to forgive others may be a reason why our prayers about other matters are not answered. See Mark 11:24-25. We need to take this statement of Jesus seriously for it may well be a cause for unanswered prayer or lack of blessing. Am I continuing to hold a grudge against someone else? If so, I need to remember that this grudge is hurting primarily me and is causing my prayers to go unanswered.

Anger, Illness, and Forgiving Others

How can we help another person forgive an offender?
1. Ask the person to describe the offending person and the event.
2. Ask him how he feels about the offender.
3. Ask him to rate on a scale of 0 to 5 the intensity of his anger or resentment.
4. Ask which person is most harmed by his anger and resentment: the one who has offended him, or he himself?
5. Now ask if he would like to get rid of the anger, resentment, and bitterness. If necessary, explain what forgiveness is and what it is not, and remind him of God's command to us to forgive others.
6. If he does want to forgive, lead him in a simple prayer releasing to God the one who has offended him, declaring to God that he is forgiving him, and asking God now to take away the bitterness and anger and replace them with his peace.

Anger at God

On page one, we asked you how you would respond to someone who was angry at God. This actually happened one day when a surgeon was doing a pre-operative evaluation of a man who needed a major operation. He asked the man about his faith in God. The man angrily replied, "How can I believe in a God who would allow a drunk driver to kill my little son?"

Many people want to blame God for the bad things that happen to them. By doing so, they want to absolve themselves of the responsibility of working through the tragedy.
Bad things happen to most of us, often for reasons we cannot determine. How can we respond to a person who expresses anger against God as this man did? This can be difficult and it requires much grace and wisdom from God to help someone through this.

The starting point is sympathy and listening. "I am so sorry to hear about that. Can you tell me about it?" Listen carefully to the story and allow the person to express the anguish, anger, and grief he has been carrying in his heart. This by itself can be very helpful to him. When he has finished the story, express empathy. "That must have been a terrible blow for you and for your family. Are you still having difficulty dealing with this tragedy?"

Do not try to defend God; he needs no defensive advocate. The grieving and angry person, however, does need help, for the bitterness and anger have negative effects on health and may diminish the ability to cope with the illness or the surgery.

Although we cannot fully understand the problem of evil and why it is so powerful and frequent, we do know that God has given us the freedom to choose our behavior. He will not take that freedom from us. We are free to do good things or bad things, but we are not free from the consequences of the things we do. These consequences affect not only us but can also affect other people. In other words, if we do something evil, this can cause suffering and even death for other people. If a man chooses to drink heavily and then drive his vehicle, God does not take those choices away from him, and others may suffer. And God did know that our freedom and the evil resulting from it would cost him the life of even his own Son.

On the other hand, we know that in all of our circumstances God is working to accomplish good things. It requires faith on our part to believe this even when we cannot imagine what good may come out of a tragedy such as the loss of a child.

Where was God when the drunk driver killed this boy? He was there, and he probably was weeping. He does not want people to abuse, kill or destroy other people. His time of judgment will come to everyone, to those who do evil and to those who do good. In the meantime, however, he can work to help us if we so choose, and he even tries to help those who do bad things in order to bring change into their lives.

God is well acquainted with the pain and anguish we suffer when others wrong us because he himself watched us kill his own Son, and he did not intervene to stop that. On the contrary, he used that heinous crime where we crucified God's Son to bring out of it eternal benefit for all who come to Jesus through faith. The God who brought eternal glory for himself and for us out of the death of his Son can also bring good out of the tragic things that happen to us if, in faith, we ask him to do so.

Helping people who are angry with God is difficult because they have a wrong understanding of God. Quietly and prayerfully explain to them the true nature of God. He gave his own Son for us in order to take away not only our sin but also the pain, anguish, bitterness, and grief from our hearts. Help them to see that
1. God is a God of comfort who can comfort us in all of our distresses.
2. He is a God of love and not of immediate retribution.
3. He is just, yet he is also patient.
4. He wants everyone to be saved from sin, from drunkenness, from abusing or killing others, and from all of the evil things we do.
5. He is always present with us even in the most difficult circumstances and he can help us cope with them if we turn to him.
6. He wants to comfort and encourage us so that we can then comfort and encourage others who are in similar circumstances.

This may speak a word of healing to the heart of someone who is angry with God.

Often in these situations forgiveness is necessary. It is not forgiveness of God, because God does no evil. Rather, it is forgiving the one who has done the evil thing. Helping a person do this can be hard, but it will be immensely healing for him if he is indeed able to release to God the one who has caused this pain.

If, however, the level of anger is so high that a person refuses to listen, then go no further in the discussion. Do not argue about the nature of God, or that God "did not kill your son," for that may cut off further dialogue. Rather, demonstrate the love of God by the loving care you give to him. Then continue to pray for the opportunity on another occasion to speak a word of healing.

<u>Two helpful books on forgiveness:</u>

Catherine Marshall: *Something More*, McGraw-Hill, New York, 1974.
   See especially chapter 3: "Forgiveness, The Aughts and the Anys", pp 35-57.
Lewis B. Smedes: *Forgive and Forget*, Harper and Row, San Francisco, 1984

Anger, Illness, and Forgiving Others

Questions for reflection
1. Describe how anger can cause physical illness.

2. List steps we should take, when angry, to control it and resolve it.

3. Describe what forgiveness really means so that you can explain it clearly to someone who truly needs to forgive an offender.

Personal questions
1. Review your own life. Make a list of those who have hurt you and whom you have not yet forgiven.

2. How can you go about forgiving them?

Homework:
Read lesson 18 in *Helping Hurting People* on Helping People Cope with Stress

Lesson 18
Helping People Who Are Carrying a Heavy Load of Stress

Stress is a normal part of life. Stress is usually not the problem unless it is excessive. The real problem is in how we respond to it. Our concern here is not to seek ways to diminish the stress on hurting people, for that is not our role. It is rather how to help them find better ways to cope with it.

Major stressors in our lives
1. Over-stimulation – too much work, family responsibilities, and so forth
2. Threats to our lives, security, goals, or happiness
3. Loss of a supporting structure

In the DVD we compare ourselves to a hot water tank capable of handling a certain level of pressure from the heat and steam. Hot water comes into the tank through an inflow pipe. It flows out from the bottom of the tank through the outflow pipe controlled by a release valve. On the top of the tank is a safety valve which can open in order to release pressure if the pressure inside the tank becomes too high. You see this in the drawing on the next page. [1]

Stress is a normal part of life just as heat is normal inside a hot water tank. Hot water tanks are built to withstand a certain level of pressure. So are we. Keeping the 'hot water' of stress flowing normally through us is essential to maintain our health, and knowing how to do that is very important. We also have various means to "let off steam," (a safety valve) in order to bring down the level of stress (pressure) in our lives. It is important that we maintain these release mechanisms so that we do not 'break' under the pressures of our life.

Warning signs of stress overload
1. Tension headaches, chronic pain, or myalgias (chronic muscle pain)
2. Chronic fatigue
3. Disturbance of sleep or disturbing dreams
4. Irritability with others and especially with family members or colleagues
5. Depression and poor ability to concentrate
6. Diminished creativity
7. Loss of a sense of humor
8. Increased dependence on TV or other distractions
9. Much time spent on the internet: games, pornography, etc.
10. Particular body symptoms, peculiar to each person

Factors that diminish our ability to handle stress
1. Too much caffeine
2. Alcohol, drugs, tobacco
3. Dependence on medications – tranquilizers, pain relievers
4. Compulsive behavior – over-eating, obsessive jogging

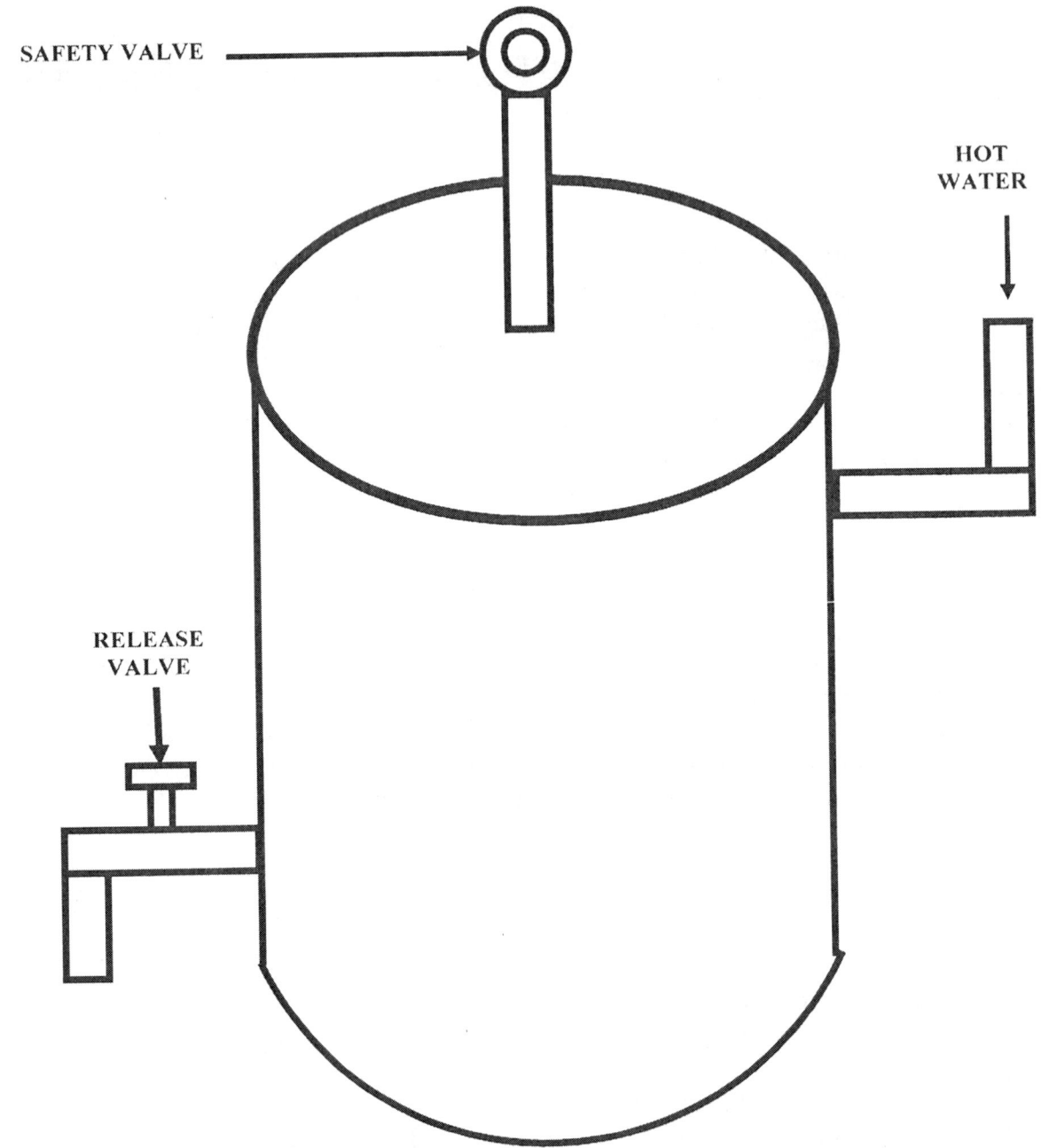

1. Adapted from Rev. Skip McCarty, Andrews University, Berrien Springs, MI

Helping a person who is stressed-out

Ask a person who has a chronic illness (which is probably a high percentage of those for whom you care): "Are you carrying a heavy load of stress?" If the answer is affirmative, then say: "Tell me about it."

Ask how things are going in their life, not just in the illness, but at home, in their marriage, with family, in their work, and so forth. Are other matters giving them worries, anxiety, or stress? If so, how are they coping with them? Ask questions like these:

Helping People Who Are Carrying a Heavy Load of Stress

1. Is all of this stress affecting your work, or sleep, or eating?
2. How are you feeling physically?
3. Are you drinking lots of coffee, tea, or other beverages with caffeine?
4. Are you taking any medicines to help you cope with it?
5. Do you have anyone to help you with this – family members, friends, a support group?
6. Has God been of help to you in this?

<u>Factors that increase our ability to handle stress</u>
1. An intimate relationship with God and dependence on his wisdom and guidance
2. Releasing cares and burdens to God regularly – I Peter 5 : 7
3. Maintaining good relations with family, friends, and associates
4. Relaxation – a good book, quiet music, fun, games
5. Exercise – regular aerobic exercise, within limits of health
6. Good nutrition – regular meals, high fiber diet low in sugar and fat, no junk food
7. Good thoughts – Philippians 4 : 8
8. Maintaining healthy attitudes
9. Making time a servant, rather than submitting to time pressure – good planning is helpful in accomplishing this
10. Being flexible, responding to unscheduled events in healthy ways

<u>Helping a person deal with on-going stress</u>

Stress comes in one of two ways, or often both together. Internal stress is the result of personal life issues, worries, or negative feelings and emotions. External stress comes from the circumstances around us: painful relationships, excessive demands, uncertainties, or violent surroundings. We can do much to work through internal stress to find resolution. However, many times external stressors cannot be changed and we can do little or nothing to diminish, eliminate, or avoid them. An old poem puts it this way:

> Lord, give me the courage to change what can be changed;
> Give me the grace to accept what cannot be changed;
> And give me the wisdom to know the difference.

How can we help people who face difficult and stressful situations every day that are impacting them negatively? How can we help them improve their coping skills?
1. A careful analysis of the stressors can help. What can be changed and how? What cannot be changed?
2. Review with the person the factors listed above that can improve one's ability to deal with stress.
3. Encourage them to find others who can be supportive of them
4. Point out biblical resources that can be of help, and resources that a close relationship with the Lord can provide. However, avoid 'throwing' verses from the Bible at them. These can become unhelpful clichés.
5. Pray with them and encourage them to develop an effective prayer strategy.

One helpful verse is in I Peter 5 : 7 where Peter says, "Cast all your care on him (Christ), for he cares for you." Here is a helpful symbol of what Jesus can do for us. Tell a hurting person to imagine the Lord standing in front of him holding a large garbage bin with the cover off. Suggest that, in prayer, he describe to the Lord the problem, or problems, and then dump them into this garbage bin. He can now imagine Christ putting the lid back on and taking the garbage bin away. He can ask the Lord to replace the worry fear, anger, or anxiety in his heart with the peace of Christ that passes our understanding.

Another helpful verse is Philippians 4 : 6 - 7

> Don't worry about anything, but in all your prayers, ask God for what you need, always asking with a thankful heart. And the peace of God, which is far beyond human understanding, will keep your heart and mind safe in union with Christ.

If the person is willing, pray together about the whole situation and commend the person and the situation into the hands of the Lord.

Helping People With Chronic Pain

Many people suffer from chronic pain – headaches, arthritis, muscle pains, neuralgias, and other conditions such as chronic fatigue syndrome or fibromyalgia. In some cases the cause of the pain is physical. In other cases the real cause is stress. In all cases, the emotional stress of the constant or recurring pain is real and can aggravate the problem of pain. Therefore, helping people deal with stress in their life can be of real benefit to them. This includes dealing not only with the stress coming from the pain, but also the stress from other current issues or problems that may have occurred in the past.

In talking with such people about stress in their lives, we must be very careful. We want to avoid any implication that their personal life is causing or aggravating the pain. It may be, but they will initially have difficulty in dealing with that. They will need to come to that realization on their own.

Describe to them how life is all put together. What happens in our lives affects our thoughts, feelings, and emotions. These in turn affect our physical body. That is how God has made us. Proverbs 14 : 30 can be useful here, especially if you sense that the person is a Christian, or is at least open to talking about what the Bible says. Once this is understood, you can explain how dealing effectively with stress can be of help in coping with the chronic pain.

On occasion, a long-standing painful illness comes from stressful events in the past, often the distant past. It may be from childhood abuse, a difficult home situation, problems with one or both parents, or something the person has done that is still causing anxiety, anger, or guilt. Looking at the picture of the heart as a home can help a person understand this better. What has happened in the past is still stored in the memory where it can continue to influence subconsciously what goes on in the "rooms" of the feelings, emotions, and desires. These in turn have an effect on physical processes – hormones, blood pressure, etc.

The 'river of life' symbol can likewise be helpful. If the hurting person seems serious in wanting to work on inner problems, describe this symbol to him and suggest that he may find it useful. Ask him if he has had problems in the past, even in childhood, that are still painful to think about. If he does identify some event, or a difficult situation, help him identify his feelings about it.

1. Is he still angry or bitter?
2. Does he need to forgive someone?

3. Does he need to ask forgiveness from the Lord?
4. Can he turn the event, the situation, or the person over to the Lord?

If he has a painful memory of trauma, abuse, fear, or confusion, when you pray with him, ask Jesus to go to that painful memory and show to him that he was there in that situation and understood the pain, fear, or confusion. Ask Christ now to take away the anguish and replace it with his peace and the assurance that he has now healed the pain of that memory. Then thank the Lord for that.

On the other hand, if he says he has no particular worries in the present, and cannot identify any painful situations in the past, don't press it. Simply pray with him (if he wishes), asking the Lord to take away the pain. Ask the Lord also to show you or the person unrecalled painful events that may be triggering the pain or condition. God occasionally reveals a suppressed but painful event or situation which, when resolved, can reduce internal stress and relieve or diminish the associated symptoms. Pray also for wisdom in knowing what else needs to be done to help him cope better with the illness.

On occasion, you will sense the person has a serious inner problem but is not yet able to talk about it. In this case, tell him you will be happy to see him again when he returns for another appointment. Keep the relationship open. Often the person will continue to think about the questions you have asked or the suggestions you have made, and later will be willing to follow through on them.

Finally, a person may have a serious problem where you feel unable to be of sufficient help. If that is the case, suggest that he consider getting help from a professional counselor. If he is open to this, see how best this can be arranged.

Helping Hurting People

Questions for reflection
1. Explain the physiological mechanisms that can cause chronic pain or fatigue.

2. List ways you can explain the links between the inner stress and the physical symptoms so that a hurting person can understand and accept this.

3. List appropriate suggestions you can make to a heavily stressed person about stress reduction.

Questions for personal reflection
1. Think back to times of painful stress in your life. How did you handle them?

2. What resources were especially helpful?

Homework
Read lesson 19 in *Helping Hurting People* on Helping a Person Face Cancer

Lesson 19
Helping A Person Face Cancer

<u>What is cancer?</u>
1. Certain cells in an organ become abnormal and escape the control of the body.
2. Normally they are destroyed by a strain of white blood cells called "killer cells."
3. If they are not destroyed, they reproduce more abnormal cells and cancer develops.
4. If our immune system is strong, we have good protection against cancer.
5. If our immune system is weak, we are more susceptible to it.

<u>General causes of cancer</u>
1. Outside substances, such as tobacco, certain food additives, radiation, etc. If we are exposed to high levels of one of these substances, too many abnormal cells are produced and the "killer cells" cannot destroy them all.
2. If the immune system is weak, the killer cells are too few or weak to destroy even the amount of abnormal cells formed regularly. We then may get cancer.

WHY DO PEOPLE GET CANCER?

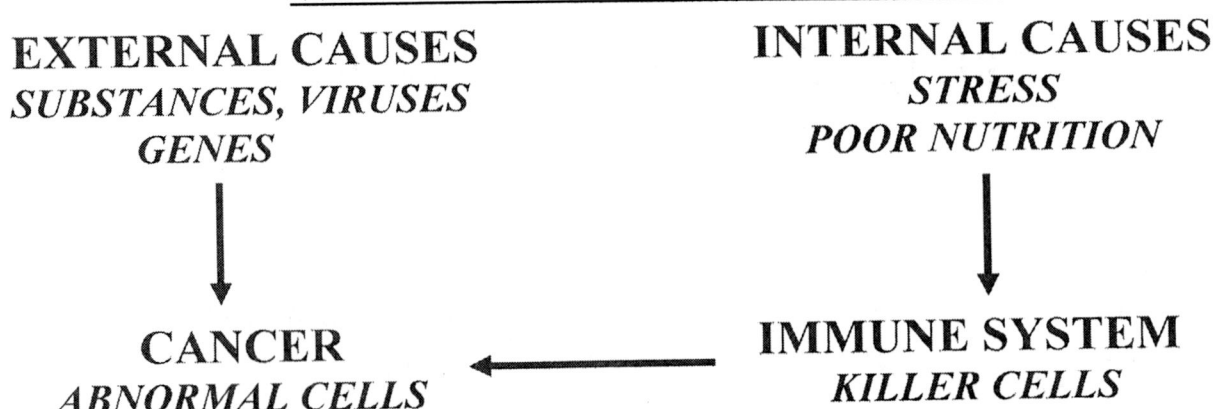

HOW DO WE TREAT CANCER?

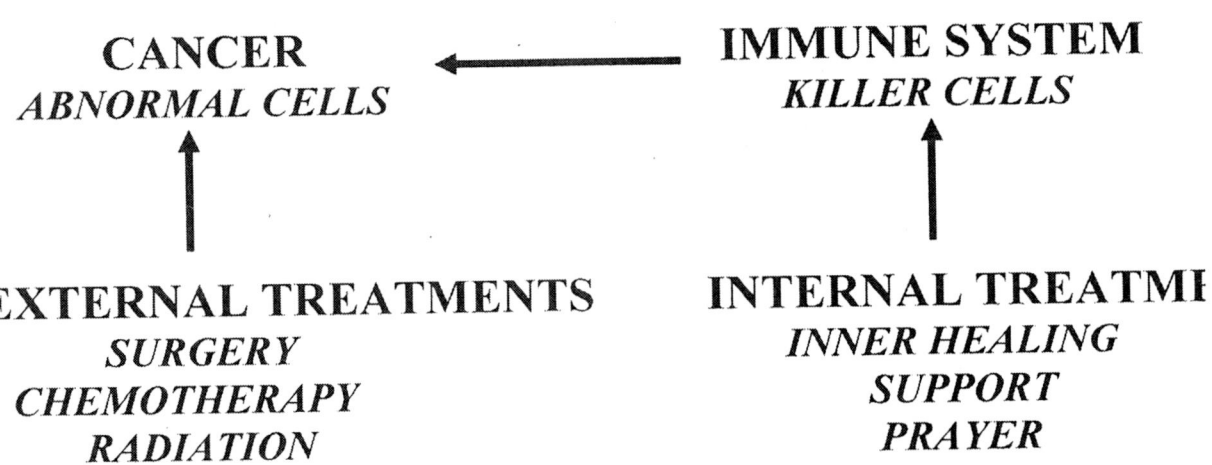

These drawings illustrate the fact that we can fight cancer on both sides of the above equation. Medical science has marvelous ways of attacking cancer cells and, in some cases, can remove them completely or retard and limit their growth.

At the same time, we can try to help the immune system of the person with cancer become stronger. More killer cells will now join the fray, and this can improve the possibilities of remission or even cure. This is why cure of the soul leading toward peace of mind can play a real role in helping persons suffering from a malignant disease.

Three types of response to cancer
1. Despair. These persons give up immediately, and the cancer progresses rapidly to death. Perhaps 10% of people diagnosed with cancer respond this way.
2. Passive acceptance. These people accept the diagnosis, allow the physicians to make all decisions, and leave the outcome to God. About 75% respond this way.
3. Fighters – 15% or more. These people take the initiative in combating the disease. They often survive much longer than expected, and many even recover completely.

If it seems appropriate, try to help those with cancer come into the third category by encouraging them to fight against their disease..

People with cancer can fight it by:
1. Reading extensively about their type of cancer and the treatments available – books, articles, and information on the internet.
2. Getting rid of any known cancer-producing agents.
3. Discussing the possible options with their physicians
4. Entering into the decision process with their physicians to decide the best and most acceptable treatment.
5. Reviewing their life. Getting relationships in order with God and with other people. Turning over burdens, concerns, and negative feelings to the Lord. This strengthens the immune system.
6. Entering into a relationship with Jesus Christ, or strengthening it. This brings peace, joy, and new meaning to life, all of which strengthen the immune system and the killer cells.
7. Trusting in God's presence and power to be with them through the whole process, working out his plan for the future, and believing it is a good plan – Isaiah 43:1-3; Jeremiah 29: 11-13
8. Focusing on constructive thoughts, feelings, and emotions. Serving others can be beneficial. So also is self-affirmation, learning to "love one's self."
9. Having a good support structure – family, friends, church, support groups.
10. Praying much – individually and with others.

In praying about cancer, it should begin by seeking God's plan and listening for his instructions. That 'still small voice' speaking to the heart is very important. Prayer for healing should be specific prayer:
1. for help in dealing with symptoms
2. for wisdom in choosing the best therapy
3. for God to increase the strength of the immune system and especially those white blood cells – "killer cells" – that fight the cancer cells

Cancer cells grow and reproduce rapidly. They require an increased amount of blood. Therefore, the blood supply to where the cancer exists increases. Here is where prayer can possibly intervene. We can ask God, who knows where all our blood vessels are, to shut down the blood vessels taking blood to the cancer cells, thus cutting off their blood supply and suffocating them.

Avoid false hopes
1. All of these measures taken together do not guarantee a cure, and we should not give the impression that they do.
2. They can improve the strength of the body and the ability to cope with the disease.
3. If recovery does not occur, we should **never** say: "It is because you have not tried hard enough, or do not have sufficient faith, or have some unconfessed sin."

Here are two excellent books about helping persons face cancer:
When God & Cancer Meet, Lynn Eib, Tyndale House, Wheaton, IL 2002
Finding the Light in Cancer's Shadow, Lynn Eib, Tyndale House, Wheaton, IL 2006

Mrs. Eib is a 'cancer victor,' and a committed Christian. She works full-time in the office of a Christian oncologist seeing every person who comes for therapy. Because of her own experience, and of a growing experience in helping hurting people, she has great insight into how to come alongside people going through the cancer experience.

Questions for reflection

1. In the etiology of cancer, what is the interaction between external and internal causal factors?

2. How can we help a person mobilize internal resistance to cancer?

3. Is there a relationship between God's healing power and our immune system?

Homework

Read lesson 20 in *Helping Hurting People* on Helping People Who Are Grieving

Lesson 20
Helping a Person Who is Grieving

"The price of love is the pain of separation."

Grieving is the result of losing someone or something to whom we are closely attached. It is the psychological pain occurring when a part of our inner self has been torn away. The deeper the attachment (love), the greater the pain of separation.

Our deepest grief comes from the loss of someone very close to us – husband or wife, child, parent, sibling, or special friend. Two lives become intimately intertwined, and then one is gone leaving a gaping hole in the heart. From this comes a real identity crisis:
- I am no longer married
- I have no one to share my sorrows and joys with.
- I have no one to touch, or to touch me.
- I will never see my loved one again.

How can we be of help to someone who is grieving such a loss?

1. Listen to the person's story. Simply listening attentively can be of immense help to a person who no longer has someone close or safe to talk to.

2. Encourage the person to talk about the one who is gone. For a new widow or widower
   - Tell me what he or she was like.
   - How long had you been married, or known one another?
   - How did you meet?
   - What did you especially enjoy doing together?

   When it is the loss of a parent, a child, or a close friend
   - Tell me what he or she was like.
   - What are some of your fondest memories?

If you can encourage a grieving person to relive some of the joys of that relationship, this can help restore a measure of peace and lead toward acceptance of the separation.

3. Ask the person what support groups he or she has – family members, church, clubs, or other people with whom to talk and develop deeper relationships and even establish new ones.

4. Inquire about activities: hobbies, creative efforts, and activities outside the home that can engage his or her interest. If it seems appropriate, suggest activities you feel might be helpful.

5. Ask about faith. Gently inquire about beliefs of life after death; of being reunited eventually in the presence of God. When the time seems right, and if the person is interested, you may want to share your personal faith about this. An understanding of the hope of eternal life is a potent antidote to despair over the loss of someone dear.

6. Help the grieving person find a purpose in the grieving. The Apostle Paul gives marvelous counsel when he says, "Praise be to the God and Father of our Lord Jesus Christ, the Father of compassion, and the God of all comfort, who comforts us in all our troubles, so that we can comfort those in any trouble with the comfort we ourselves have received from God (II Corinthians 1:3–4 NIV). If you have been through grieving because of the loss of a loved one, you can share how the lessons you learned in that process enable you now to bring help to others.

7. Lesson 15 on helping a person find happiness and purpose in life may be of help. Talk about developing new relationships, of the benefits of reaching out to serve others, and of deepening a relationship with God.

8. Acceptance of the loss is an important but difficult step. It comes slowly but can be encouraged with help. Helping the grieving person understand the change in self-identity and trying to discover a new purposeful identity can be of benefit.

9. Prayer is important, if accepted. A quiet sincere prayer where you ask for the comfort and presence of God and the reassurance of the goodness of life can speak words of comfort to the bereaved.

Many who come to you in a time of bereavement will be helped by these measures. Often you will need to say very little. The assurance of being a good listener and a faithful friend in whom the person can trust will bring relief and release to many.

Be attentive to the emotional expressions of the grieving person. Weeping is normal. Tears are the means by which we express grief and act as 'organs of elimination' of the grief. Be patient when a person weeps. Wait quietly until he or she can again talk with you. A gentle touch of the hand may be appropriate. Keep a box of facial tissue handy.

Watch for signs of protracted or abnormal grief:
- a duration that seems to long
- loss of affect or a sense of humor
- inability to concentrate
- loss of appetite
- insomnia

If you feel a grieving person is in danger of a deep or morbid depression, professional help may be necessary for the person.

Helping a Person Who is Grieving

Questions for reflection
1. Have you been through a period of intense grieving yourself?

2. What resources did you find that were helpful to you?

3. What are indications that the person is handling the grief normally?

4. What are indications of abnormal grieving?

Homework
Read lesson 21 on Helping People Cope with Bad News and Terminal Illness

Lesson 21
Helping People Cope with Bad News and Terminal Illness
God, Medicine, and Miracles, chapter 12

Bad news comes to all of us at one or more times in our lives. Our response to it depends on several factors:
1. The nature of the problem
2. How the news came to us
3. Available social support structures
4. How strong we are in our spirit to be able to deal with it.

Helping people who have received bad news

Many times people come to us having already received the bad news. Our concern in this situation is to help them find strength and ways to respond to it constructively. Find out as much about the situation as the sick person is willing to tell you, but without putting any pressure on him or her. Is it:
- A bad diagnosis; a threatening prognosis?
- A difficult treatment?
- A serious loss?

Reflect the person's feelings by a statement like:
- You must be afraid…..worried……deeply concerned…..very sad

You could ask:
- How is this going to affect your life? your family? your plans, hopes, dreams?

This is often an occasion to discuss faith:
- Tell me about your faith.
- Is your faith being of help to you in this?
- How are you praying about this?

Telling bad news to people

On other occasions we are the ones who have to tell bad news to people. It may be the diagnosis of a life-threatening illness, like cancer or HIV/AIDS. It may be the need for a difficult treatment – amputation, or a dangerous procedure. In this case, we must know how to convey the bad news in a way that is gentle, clear, and offers hope.

Hope

Hope is an essential ingredient for life and for daily living. Even in the face of a seemingly fatal prognosis, there can always be hope for:
1. eternal life
2. meaning and purpose during the remaining days (years) of life
3. peace and strength to cope with the situation
4. for a possible remission
5. and sometimes for a successful treatment

Assessment of strengths

Ask the person about his or her accomplishments in the past. "What have you done that has succeeded well?" Then inquire about how the person handled the challenges, opportunities, and difficulties of the task, and how he or she overcame the obstacles. In this way you can challenge the person to bring these strengths and assets to bear in dealing with the current situation. The past challenge may have been
- in the military
- in business
- in raising a fine family
- a major sports event
- a hunting expedition
- something else related to a major life interest

Try to help the person mobilize the courage and resourcefulness used to cope with the past challenges to cope now with the current problem. Encourage the person to find out as much as possible about the disease or the treatment, and to look into the options. Armed with this information, the person can then discuss the options with the caregivers and be involved in the decision-making process. Being actively involved in one's treatment and in the whole healing process is of great benefit.

Here are some guidelines for presenting difficult news with compassion and gentleness
1. Lead up to the bad news slowly and carefully. Never be abrupt: "You have cancer." or "Your test for AIDS is positive." That borders on brutality.
2. Emphasize what can be done medically to help mitigate the situation.
3. Offer psychological and spiritual encouragement and point out the resources God makes available to us to strengthen us inwardly.
4. Assure the person of the on-going support of the health caregivers.
5. Encourage the person to mobilize family and other social supports structures to accompany him or her on this journey.
6. Offer prayer.

Read Norman Cousins' classical book: *The Anatomy of an Illness as Perceived by the Patient.* Cousins describes how he coped with a rapidly progressive, painful, and seemingly fatal disease. He focused on positive thoughts and concentrated on helpful emotions such as joy and laughter. The disease process gradually and completely abated, his strength returned, and within a year he recovered. Sharing this story or recommending the book to someone with a serious illness can be helpful.

Trust in God

When a difficult circumstance comes and worry, grief, or fear occur, we can step back momentarily, focus on God, and ask God how we should respond. Romans 8 : 28 assures us God is at work in all of our circumstances for our good. This does not imply that:

- God sends these circumstances, although he has allowed them to happen.
- God intends to "fix" them. He does not give us immunity from difficult circumstances, but he does promise to accompany us through them.
- It does mean, however, that God is able to work in and through them to help us to grow in wisdom, in spiritual maturity, and in trust.

To learn to trust God takes time and effort, but it is worth it. Suggest to the person
1. Keep remembering to consult with God regularly, even many times a day.
2. Keep emotions under control.
3. Learn more about God and the life he wants us to live. This comes primarily from God's Word.
4. Commit his or her life and circumstances to God's control, then discern from him how best to respond.

Helping Hurting People

Questions for reflection

1. List the principles we should follow in giving bad news to a hurting person.

2. What coping resources can we suggest to them?

3. In what ways can we convey hope to them?

Helping People Cope with Bad News and Terminal Illness

Caring for Persons Who Are Terminally Ill

Emotional problems

Severe illness with the possibility of death in the near future brings many difficult feelings and emotions.
1. Denial: "It can't be true. I have lived a good life. This illness is not serious. It will soon go away. I will recover."
2. Grief: "I am going to lose my family, my work, all I had hoped to accomplish."
3. Anger: "Why is this happening to me? Why don't people help me? Is God angry with me? Why doesn't he heal me?"
4. Fear: "What is going to happen to me? Where will I go?"
5. Shame: "This illness is stronger than I am. I can't overcome it. I am losing the battle."
6. Resignation: "There is nothing I can do. It is my fate (or God's will). So be it!"
7. Bargaining, or self-help: "If I can just do what God wants me to do, I will get better."
8. Depression: "I give up. I have no energy or desire to try to recover or get stronger. It is finished for me."

These feelings are in the heart as the thought of death is in the mind. Because of this, it is difficult for a dying person to talk openly about the possibility of death. As we care for severely ill persons, we should try to discern if any of these difficult feelings are present. If so, fear of death or despair may keep them from talking. Yet it can be of great benefit to dying persons to have someone who will listen to them and in whom they can put their confidence. We should therefore look for opportunities to help a person begin to express these difficult feelings and emotions.

If the sick person raises the question of possible death, it is because he is reaching out for help. This gives us an opportunity to sit with him, listen to his concerns, and share hope with him. Other times, however, a person is afraid to discuss the severity of his own illness or the possibility of dying. By keeping the painful emotions inside, he is increasing his suffering. How can we help such a person?

The starting point is to become acquainted with the person and build a relationship of confidence. We can do this as we spend time with him, listening to anything he may say, and giving compassionate care. Once a relationship of confidence has been established, we can ask open questions such as:
1. How are you really feeling?
2. Are you worried about your condition?
3. Are you afraid of what might happen to you?

These questions give the person an opportunity to express his concerns and worries if he wishes to do so. He may describe his fear of the future and even of dying. If so, we can proceed further. If he does not seem able to bring up the subject of possible death, we can then ask:
1. Are you afraid you might die of this illness?
2. If so, are you afraid to die?

Once the subject of death has been brought up and discussed, we can proceed along these lines.

1. Explain that death is an event that will come to all of us. It is helpful to think about it ahead of time. We can then prepare for it, and we can help our families prepare for it.
2. Then ask: From you own faith, what do you believe will happen when you die? Where will you go?

Listen carefully to the response. If the person has the assurance of eternal life through faith in Christ, reinforce this. Talk about the anticipated joys of being in the presence of God and being reunited with loved ones.

If the dying person has no assurance of eternal life, we must try to help him with this. What follows here, about other religions, is a brief summary to help you. It is not necessary to discuss this with most persons. You may, however, have the opportunity to care for someone of one of the other major religions, so keep in mind what follows.

Almost all religions believe that physical death is a transition into another state of being. It is not the end of everything. Rather, it means leaving the current existence and state of consciousness and going somewhere else.

Hindus and Buddhists believe that a person is reborn into another life, either human or animal. The form into which one is reborn depends on the accumulated merit, or "karma" in this life. There is no certain way of knowing what merit has been accumulated, or whether the next "life" will be better or worse than the present one. So the person faces an unknown situation.

In Islam, Muslims believe that a person comes into the presence of Allah who will then judge what the next existence is to be like. Allah judges on the basis of the merit the person has accumulated in this life, and his judgment is final. One can never be certain what the judgment of Allah will be, even though efforts have been made to accumulate much merit in this life.

In animistic or traditional tribal worldviews, people believe that the spirit departs to the dwelling place of spirits and will wander with the spirits of deceased family and ancestors. No certain abode is known.

<u>An open and gentle approach</u>

On pages 87 and 88 we discussed how to help a person come into a personal relationship with Christ if he or she so wishes. Talk gently with people about this, especially those who are very sick. We should put no pressure on a person to accept Christ. This must be entirely her decision. Our role is simply to explain clearly what options are available to her and what faith in Christ means and how to enter into it. Then we let the person decide. If she does decide to accept Christ and has never done that before, we can then proceed as outlined on pages 87 - 88.

Here is a helpful symbol of salvation. When we travel from one country to another, we need a passport from our own country with a visa in it to permit us to enter the new country. If we do not have a passport with the visa stamped in it, we will not be allowed to enter the new country.

God has given us all a "passport," which is our identity in our life here on earth. As our name is written clearly in our passport, so God knows our name and our identity, even those who themselves do not know God. The "visa" we need in order to live forever with God in heaven is faith in Jesus Christ. Our entrance into heaven does not depend on merit we have accumulated, or good works we have done. It depends simply on what Christ has done for us and our acceptance of that and faith in Him.

Explaining to a dying person that there is a real hope for new life can be very helpful. Hope is an essential element for our lives, and hope for eternal life is available to everyone.

Another important issue is that of preparation. Before leaving on a long journey, we prepare for the trip. It is far more important to prepare adequately for this final trip. This means arranging many affairs:
1. will
2. property and personal belongings
3. relationships

We can gently ask a person what preparations he or she has made for this coming journey. Relationships may need to be restored, and we can help them see how to do this in a God-honoring way. Explain how important it is that the family knows the wishes of the person in regard to what is being left behind. This is a real gift a dying person can give to the family, for it enables the family to work through the final arrangements and affairs with peace.

Helping Hurting People

Questions for reflection

1. What thoughts do you have about your own mortality? You may find it helpful to write them out for your own reflection. Until we are comfortable with our own mortality, it is difficult to help others facing end-of-life issues.

2. When you think about eternity, what comes to mind?

3. How should you proceed when someone tells you that he or she has just been informed of a fatal prognosis?

Homework

Read lesson 22 in *Helping Hurting People* – the final lesson, on Practical Applications

Lesson 22
Practical Applications

We have worked hard together to lay the foundation of principles and skills needed for this team approach to caring for people as whole persons. We must now look at practical issues in how to put this approach into effective use.

No one model will fit every situation, and many adaptations will need to be made according to the type of practice or clinical setting. Our experience has been in a small private clinical setting in which the whole staff plays an active role in this approach. This approach is sufficiently flexible that it can be adapted to other practice situations. It can even be implemented in a hospital or emergency room environment provided that the administrative staff is in agreement. Whatever the situation, certain principles are important, and we will take a look at them here.

Under one roof
Ideally care for body, soul, and spirit should take place in one clinical setting. This has the marvelous advantages of convenience for the sick person, regular contacts between all the members of the team, and a sense of coordination of care. Spiritual care can be given elsewhere, in a church facility or in a neutral setting somewhere else. This means, however, a separate time and place for the spiritual care.

Free of charge
This important aspect of whole person care should be free of charge. Charging a separate fee for spiritual care adds further to the financial burden of those coming for care and may prove to be an obstacle for some people. It also raises difficult legal issues. For the most part, spiritual caregivers are volunteers who give part-time service to help hurting people. As such they cost the medical service almost nothing, and their services can be offered to those who wish them without additional costs.

A separate consultation room
Spiritual care is highly personal. Privacy and the assurance of confidentiality are essential. Talking with people in a waiting room, or a break room, or some other public area can be useful. This ambiance, however, does not permit in-depth discussions about personal or family issues. Hopefully, any medical service applying this approach to whole person care will be able to provide a separate room for spiritual care. Ideally it should be furnished in a homelike fashion – comfortable furniture, a casual atmosphere, perhaps even a microwave, tea kettle for hot drinks, or even a small refrigerator. And always a box of facial tissues!

A team spirit
A close working relationship between all of the caregivers and staff – the physicians and other providers, the spiritual caregivers, members of the administrative staff – greatly facilitates the effectiveness of this approach. We would suggest a brief meeting and time of prayer for the whole team at

the beginning of the morning or afternoon, and a regular schedule when the staff and caregivers can meet to discuss any questions or issues related to this approach. Sharing experiences can be of much encouragement, although it must respect matters of confidentiality.

Confidentiality

We have discussed this throughout the course, and it is absolutely essential. We must maintain an atmosphere that is completely 'safe,' where people will be at ease to tell their personal story. It is important for us to remember that the story they tell belongs to them. It does not belong to us. We therefore have no right to pass their story on to other people unless, of course, they give explicit permission for us to do so. As we mentioned earlier, there are legal limits to confidentiality. When we discern that a person may be in a position to harm himself or herself, or another person, we are then required to pass that information on to those responsible in our service.

Keeping records

For legal purposes, we keep minimal records about the spiritual care offered. In some practices, a simple register is maintained that contains simply
- the date of each interview
- two initials of the person coming for spiritual care
- the particular issue or issues discussed
- the care offered, including prayer
- a brief note of the response
- the initials of the caregiver

However, for your personal use, learning, and growth in experience, you may want to write a more extensive note for your own private use. You can then feel free to include more details of the story each person shares with you. This can help you
- remember the events discussed if the person returns to see you
- learn from your experiences

You must keep this record strictly for yourself and in a safe place where no one else has access to it. It would be best not to include the full name of the person in each account. Since this is your own private record, no one should know about it, and it would not be a legal document that could be 'discovered' by the legal system.

Personal Bible study

We would strongly encourage you to dig deeply into the Scriptures to learn all you can about the Lord, about human life with all its problems, and about the marvelous stories and counsel we find in God's Word concerning health and healing. We suggested in an earlier lesson that you study in-depth the healing stories of Jesus – how he healed the whole person in each situation. You will notice that his approach differed in each situation, according to the person and the needs and situation of that person. You may want to do this study in a group with other caregivers or other friends of like mind. In this way you can learn from each other.

Practical Applications

Prayer

In a ministry of this nature, prayer is a great resource, and we had a whole lesson on prayer. Pray daily about your involvement in this work, and especially as you begin each period of service. Pray also for the team of which you are a member. Pray for those who have come to you for help that the power of God will continue to work in them for healing.

You may want to ask a few close friends to become partners with you in this ministry by praying for you on a daily basis and especially during the times you will be serving. A support base of real intercessors can make a major difference in the effectiveness of your caregiving.

Church support

Be sure the pastor and other leaders of your church are aware of what you are doing and are supporting you in this. At the same time, you can encourage them to become more aware of the healing power of God and of the abundant teaching in the Bible about health and healing. You may wish to encourage your church to develop an active ministry of teaching on health and healing and becoming involved in a church-based ministry of helping hurting people. Remind your church leaders that Christ gave the mandate to heal the sick to the whole church, not just to specialists.

Nervousness

Is it normal to feel nervous as you begin this ministry? Absolutely! It is very normal. You will be meeting new people. You will often be listening to difficult situations. And you may feel inadequate to be of help in some situations. One purpose of the various times of role playing throughout the training process has been to help you to become used to talking with another person about personal issues. Doing this in a perfectly safe, learning, and often fun environment has hopefully prepared you to begin this ministry.

Remember, you are not involved in this ministry alone. First of all, you are part of a team, and that team should include friends who pray regularly for you. Secondly, you are never alone, for the Lord himself is with you and will be working in each contact, interview, and helping consultation. In our experience we have often been amazed at how the Lord seems to match up the person in need and the one giving spiritual care. Many caregivers report with some excitement how they sensed the Spirit of God intervening in conversations to provide bridges of understanding and enabling the caregivers to find the resources needed by a particular person.

Moments of silence will come, and they can be beneficial. Learn to relax and wait. This can allow a hurting person to share more of a personal concern or to open up another issue for which he or she needs help. You can pray silently that the Lord will be at work in this whole process.

Long-term relationships

Some practices allow and even encourage sick persons to return to see a spiritual caregiver without a separate appointment and without necessarily seeing the health provider at the same time. This has the advantage of permitting a closer and more continuous caring relationship with a hurting person. A word of caution is in order here, however. Some people may become overly dependent on a prolonged relationship with you, and this may be unhealthy for them and for you. If you sense that such a relationship is not in the best interests of them or of you, discuss this with your health provider. It may be time to diminish or even terminate the relationship to avoid the development of a co-dependent situation.

People with chronic illnesses

In previous lessons we stressed that personal, emotional, and social factors play an important role in many chronic illnesses. This includes diseases of the heart and blood vessels, such as high blood pressure, coronary artery disease, and heart failure. It also includes adult diabetes, those with chronic pain or fatigue, certain malignancies, life-style related problems, and what we call the auto-immune diseases like certain types of asthma, arthritis, allergies, lupus, and so forth. Stress is an important component in these illnesses whether the stress comes simply from the disease itself or from personal aspects of the person's life.

Pay close attention as you listen to persons with a chronic illness like one of these. Are there family problems, painful relationships, anger, grudges, or deep resentments? Are there feelings of guilt, of shame, or of regrets for past events or deeds? Is there a significant level of fear? What is the self-esteem of a person with a chronic illness – how does he feel about himself?

If you discover a significant area of stress or an inner burden, call to mind the resources we have discussed that could be of help. Explaining gently these resources and describing how the person can make a personal application of them can be very beneficial. Prayer, of course, is of great importance, but be sure you always ask permission before you pray.

Here is where making note of each consultation with a person who has a chronic illness can be very useful. As you talk with more people with chronic illnesses, you may observe certain trends or patterns relating particular stressors to certain illnesses. If you do see such a pattern, by all means discuss it with your health provider, for this can provide information for improved care of such persons.

Culture war

In our current North American culture, pressure is increasing on the Christian community and all that is associated with churches. We must be prepared to deal with any opposition that is expressed in this regard. We have mentioned several times in previous lessons that we have a strong base of scientific evidence to support spiritual care. We likewise have evidence that specifically Christian resources are of benefit for health and for the healing of many illnesses. We can, therefore, speak clearly, though gently, about the foundation on which we stand. And we can recount the growing practical experience that is demonstrating the positive effects of this ministry.

Keep in mind the wonderful counsel of the Apostle Peter in his first letter: "Be ready at all times to explain the reason for the hope within you, but do it always with gentleness and respect" (I Peter 3 : 12). The truth is the best proponent we have, and simply describing what is happening may be our best offense in this cultural war. Keep in mind also that those expressing opposition may have deep problems within their own lives driving them to this opposition. So listen to them carefully and see if you can offer them a quiet word of encouragement to explore the reality of spiritual life through Christ.

A final word

We have come to the end of these lessons on caring for the whole person. It has been our pleasure to have worked with you on this, either directly or indirectly, and we do hope these lessons have been of use to you. We will be happy to hear from you directly or through your instructor about your evaluation of this course and if you feel that it has, or has not, been of practical help to you in preparing you for this ministry.

The real evaluation of the course, however, will come in the days ahead, as you apply these principles and skills. Feel free to contact us as you proceed in this important ministry. We will be delighted to learn of your experiences and will do what we can to be of further help to you. May the peace of the Lord be with you.

Sherry O'Donnell, D.O.

Dan Fountain, M.D., MPH

Bibliography

God, Medicine, and Miracles – Dan Fountain, Harold Shaw Publishers, 1999, WaterBrook Press, Colorado Springs, ISBN 0-87788-321-1
A discussion of the brokenness of the biomedical model, the biblical and scientific perspectives on wholeness, how Jesus heals the whole person, emotional problems that influence health, and how Jesus, by healing mind, soul, and spirit, can bring healing resources to physical health.
Much personal experience and anecdotes of healing.

Health, the Bible and the Church – Dan Fountain, Billy Graham Center, 1989, EMIS Box 794, Wheaton, IL 60189-0794 or emis@wheaton.edu
A comparison of the biblical and secular world views concerning health and health care, and a discussion of cross-cultural understanding and communication related to health issues.

The Faith Factor, Dale Matthews, Viking Press, 1998 – ISBN 0-670-87539-2
Written by a Christian professor of internal medicine. It analyzes the voluminous medical literature that documents major influences of extrinsic religion and intrinsic faith on physical health. The author believes that, because of the documented influence of religion on physical health, it is now not only ethical to discuss matters of faith and religion in the clinic but is also unethical not to do so.

The Link Between Religion and Health, Harold Koenig and Harvey Cohen of Duke, Oxford, 2002 – ISBN 0-19-514360-4
Another book laying out the observational and biomedical evidence of the important roles that stress has on health and the positive benefits of religion and faith in enabling people to cope better with stress and thus improve their health

The Anatomy of an Illness as Perceived by the Patient, Norman Cousins, W. W. Norton, New York, 1979
A story of how a man with a seemingly fatal illness recovered by taking charge of his situation and focusing on positive emotions and humor. This book helped stimulate the development of psychoneuroimmunology.

Also by Norman Cousins:
 The Healing Heart, Norman Cousins, W. W. Norton, New York, 1983
 Head First, The Biology of Hope, Norman Cousins, Penguin Books, New York, 1989

Authority to Heal, Ken Blue, IVP, Downers Grove IL, 1987. ISBN 0-8308-1700-X
Ken Blue is a leader in renewing the ministry of the church in healing. He discusses God's will for health, that God does not inflict people with illnesses for their spiritual benefit, and that it is not our faith that heals us but God's power. God makes many faith resources available to us for healing. He discussed how churches can play a much more active role in the ministry of healing.

Timeless Healing – The Power and Biology of Belief, Herbert Benson, Fireside, New York, 1996. ISBN 0-684-83146-5
Dr. Benson draws on his 25 years as a physician and researcher at Harvard to reveal how affirming beliefs, particularly belief in a higher power, make an important contribution to our physical health. He believes the majority of physical illnesses are reflections of deep-seated psycho-social problems, and that beliefs and particularly 'remembered wellness' and the 'relaxation response' can be of great benefit. He affirms faith in God, but his spirituality is quite 'generic.'

The Stress of Life, Hans Selye, McGraw-Hill, Inc., New York, 1984
A very readable summary of the research on the effects of stress on the physical body.

How to Be a People Helper, Gary R. Collins, Tyndale House Publishers, Wheaton, IL 1995
A good book on the caring relationship and how to establish an open and safe atmosphere with hurting people.

Spiritual Care, Judith Allen Shelly, InterVarsity Press, Downers Grove, 2000.
Another good book on the caring relationship

Copies of this manual may be obtained from:
Peeke School of Christian Mission
King College
1350 King college Road
Bristol, TN 37620
Phone: 423-652-4157
E-mail: globalhealth@king.edu